Silk On Ice

The Process of Growing into Grace

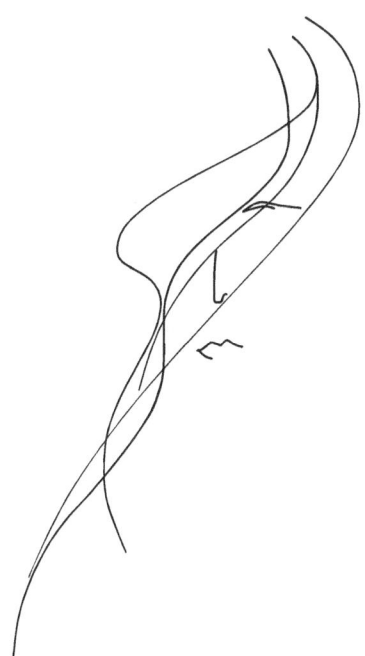

Sian Flanagan

Silk On Ice:
The Process of Growing into Grace

2024 YGTMedia Co. Press Trade Paperback Edition.
Copyright © 2024 Sian Flanagan

Published in Canada, for Global Distribution by YGTMedia Co. www.ygtmedia.co
For more information email: info@ygtmedia.co

ISBN trade paperback: 978-1-998754-59-5
ISBN hardback: 978-1-998754-61-8
ISBN eBook: 978-1-998754-60-1

To order additional copies of this book:
info@ygtmedia.co

Silk On Ice

The Process of Growing into Grace

Written and Illustrated by
Sian Flanagan

Acknowledgments

To you, my reader. Thank you for choosing
to spend your time digesting these pages.
Without you, this book is nothing more than
naked paper clothed in ink. You are my inspiration,
my reason for bringing this book to life.

An acknowledgment to Ian Macdonald:
thank you for your generosity.

For my grandmother, Grace, who has always
been a fierce lightning bolt in my life.

Contents

Stolen

surviving storms

Lay words down gently
be *silk on ice*
paint ink in spaces
that yearn for life,
play with words
that beg to be heard,
leave a piece of yourself
on every page
through letters and verbs
now go —
be fire again in flames
that burn
glow

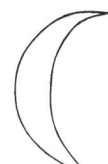

Rest assured
grace wrote this for you —
for every woman who forges on
in the face of fear

rest assured
these words are for the souls
who have strength
and unwavering courage to choose
who they want to be
for themselves and humanity

rest assured
you are brilliant
as you come
and as you go

know you are blessed
with a divine gift
every moment of this lifetime

the gift
— is you

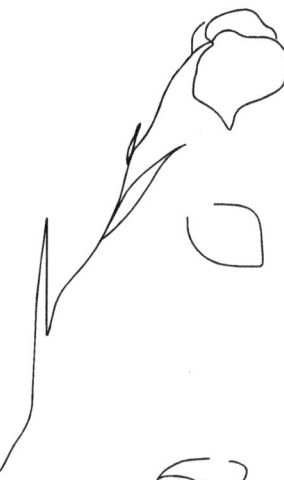

as a creator
there is always a space
within you
to navigate and feel safe
along your journey

rest assured
your innate grace
is your mother of wisdom
and you,
as you are
in any moment,
can create your world,
for your essence
is genetically coded,
you are written with wonder,
you are abundantly
imbued with love

let your heart
fly like a dove
beyond the cage
you have known
so you can grow
into a life
your soulful self
calls home

Why do you stand so firm?
because I have fallen
from this earth
so many times before

— grounded

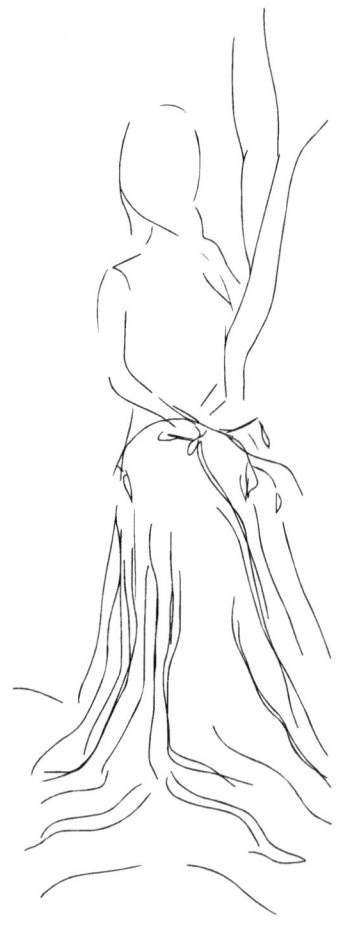

silk on ice

How long will it take to escape?
there are no shortcuts
begin the climb
each day ...

Collapsing
this house
falls inwards on itself

a pliable heart
crashes hard like
books off shelves

my ill sick slumber
keeps me locked
dawn till dusk
what brought me up
now tears me down

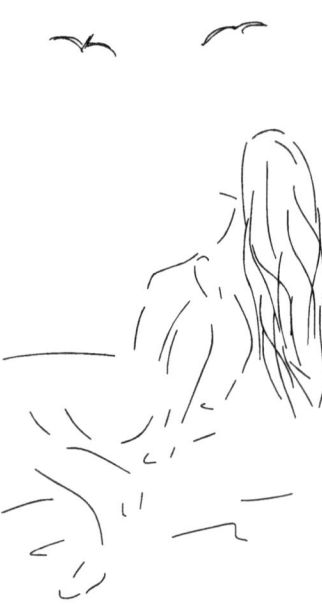

my insides exposed
a vulture's feast
bleeding through paralysis
this viscous flow
could not
move slower

The weighted vest of worry
holds many hearts down,
thoughts run wild
from radio sounds

the burden thickens
tending to dead weeds
of the past,
teaching our hearts to
hold on to the aftermath

tell me ...
what garden can grow
with seeds that lay dead?

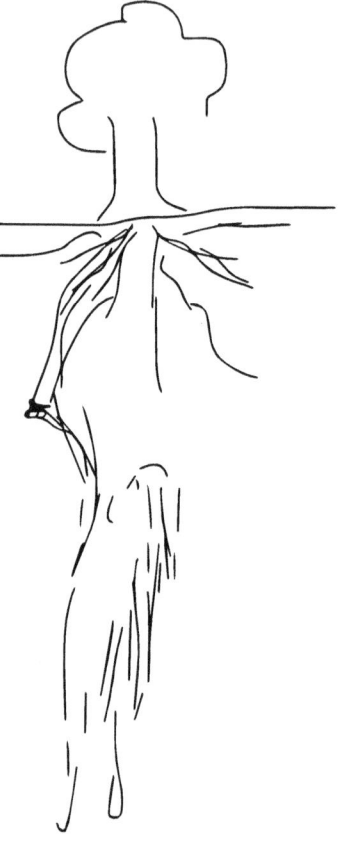

Holding on to every word
leaves us hanging on
by a thread

— projections

Tying,
collecting
rusty words from tongues
placing them high on pedestals

rehearsing beliefs
that make you weak,
blinding intuition from
where you seek to see ...

walls will always
barricade the truth
from who you are
at the root

never mute
the vines
that bear
one-of-a-kind
real fruit

Fear
led me astray
onto paths born for decay ...
do not waste time
losing life to years
navigating the journey
with the compass of fear,
life is too short for that

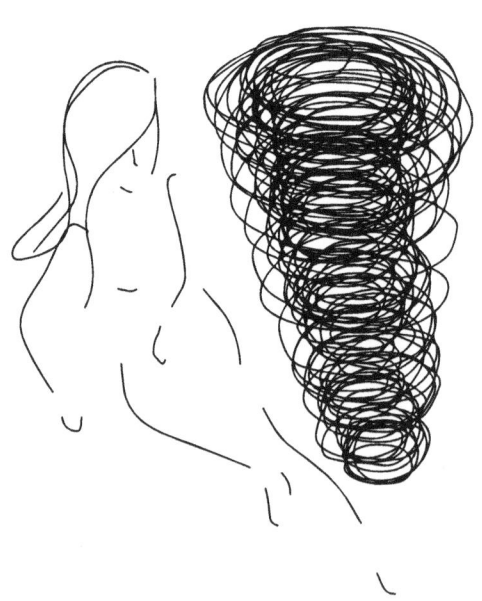

To be without grace
brings dis-ease,
unnerving,
the edge hardens

a slippery slope
destined
for self-abandonment

No one deserves
broken promises
but life happens
thoughts change
plans can form
and then run away

— shattered dreams

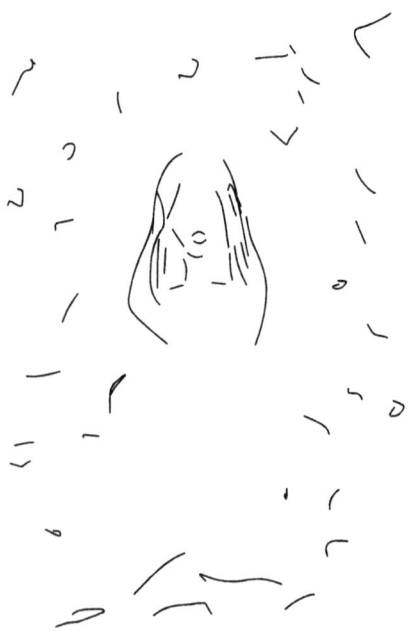

silk on ice

Panic set in

sail's too frail

to face the storm

too young,

too naive,

wrestling an ocean of words ...

there *she* lay capsized

in a world overturned

Living in negativity,
repeating words
that peel back flesh
— flayed
like Bartholomew
crucifixion
is not the way

— negative self-talk

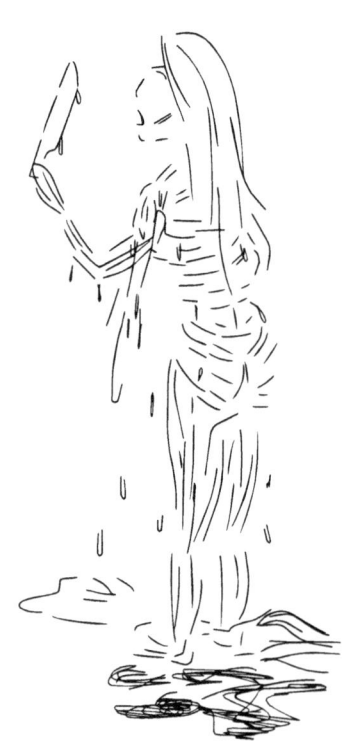

silk on ice

Thoughts torment
the needle of my thread
as I attempt to stitch
my life back
together again

— setbacks

Placing thoughts
on boomerangs
expecting them
to disappear

— anxiety

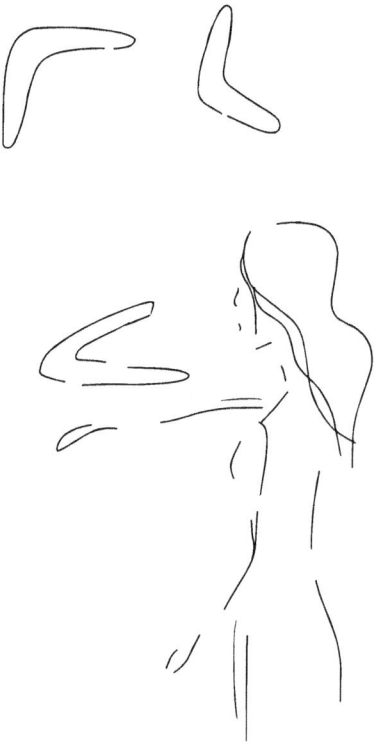

We condemn ourselves

and each other

for universal experiences

— mental dis-ease

Staring eye to eye
steam blurs my reflection

too afraid to love
who I cannot escape,
believing the world needs me
to be everything,
except who
I was designed
to be ...

mirror mirror
on the wall
casting spells
on my heart,
I yearn to see
my true reflection
beyond this hollow space,
living inside the dark

— body image

silk on ice

Purging failure
and shame
never tasted
so cruel

Is she > or = to me
Is she < or > than me
Is she < or = to me
Or are we simply =

— comparison

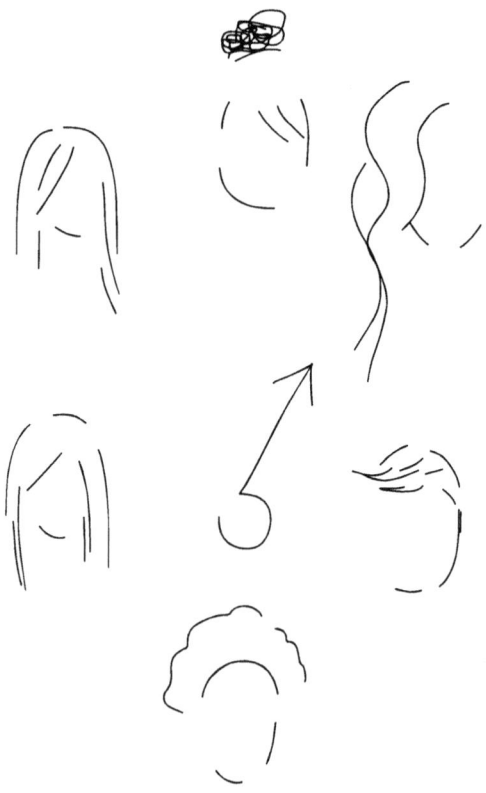

silk on ice

Weighed and measured
nails point like daggers
tipping the scale
with things
that do not matter

judgment,
comparison,
erosion chips away,
handling words
is a dangerous game

Society said:
sticks and stones
would break my bones
but words could never hurt me

yet words told stories
the kind I did not want to read
and believing them
caused my soul to bleed,
drinking the venom
they handed me,
damned in thought
depression took the lead

Neurotics endorse

the same narcotic,

voting for negativity's plague

keeps great minds at bay

Are you in there?
I need you now
more than ever

— lost

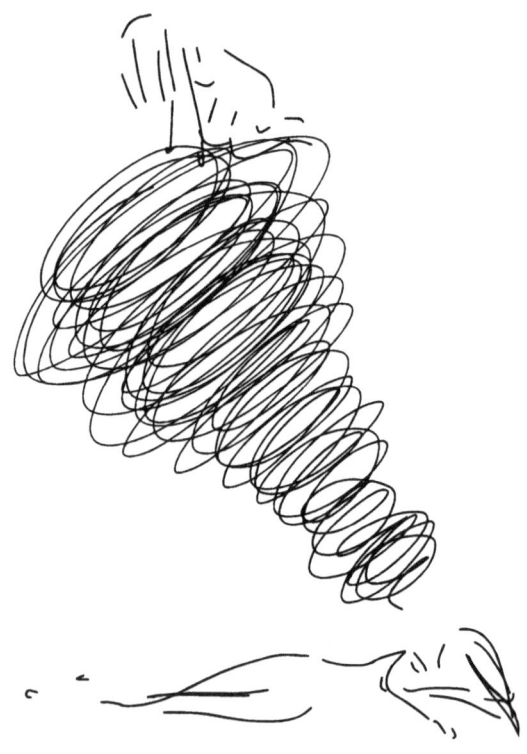

A fragile glow
grows dim with fear

black bed of cold
holds me near

this dark angel's cave
steals my nights

this feverish chill
wrestles my bones
making me ill inside

The world is waiting
patiently for you

come out of that hole
you were not born for darkness
my love

— rock bottom

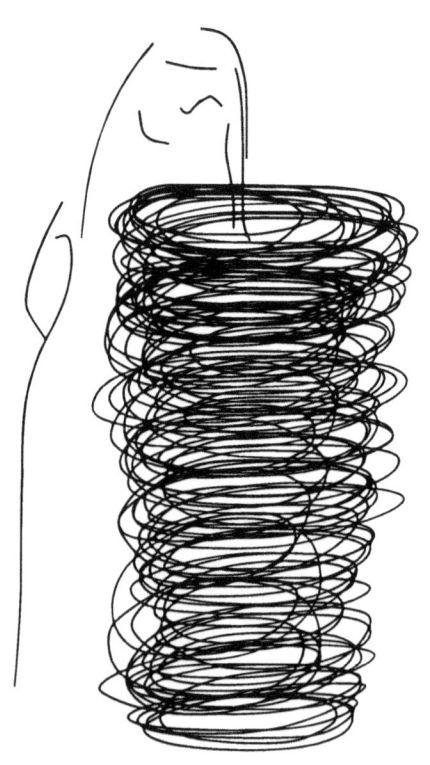

He said: I love you

And instead of knowing
how to love back,
she wrote a check
for every ounce
of self-worth she had

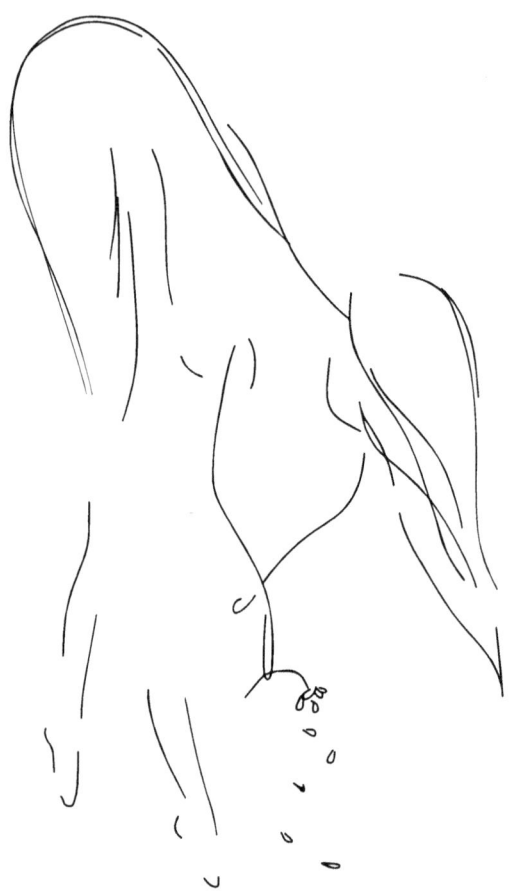

Wilting has become
of what once bloomed

— misalignment

Petals shrivel,

time grows brittle

— melting with sinking snow

this season takes me

everywhere but home

Caught
in the matrix
it guts me dry

addicted to finding pleasure
outside these walls,
comes from abiding
by society's lies

— survival mode

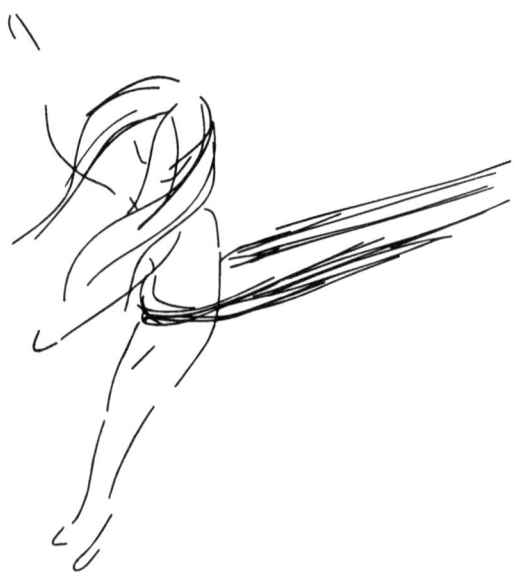

silk on ice

I am attempting
to catch myself
before I fall
and starve in oblivion

Naked armor
shed this skin
dilute the venom
that keeps my ego fed

— self-sabotage

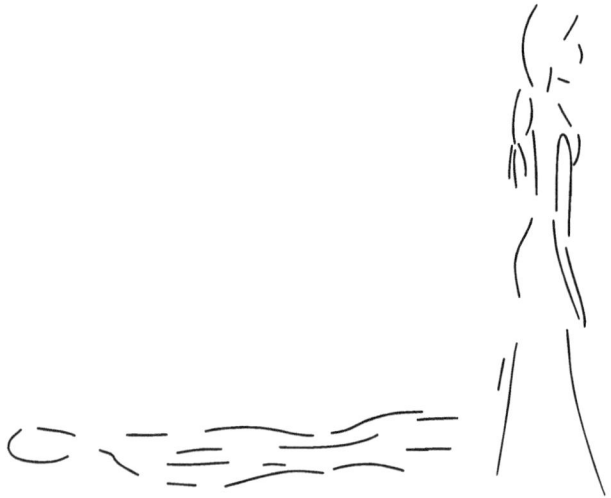

silk on ice

Shallow heart

I watch vanity brew,

frayed wires

the illusion

— is slowly invading you

You never see a traitor
until you are staring down
the barrel of their gun,
wondering how you could
have been so blind
to love someone
so much
it kills you

— betrayal

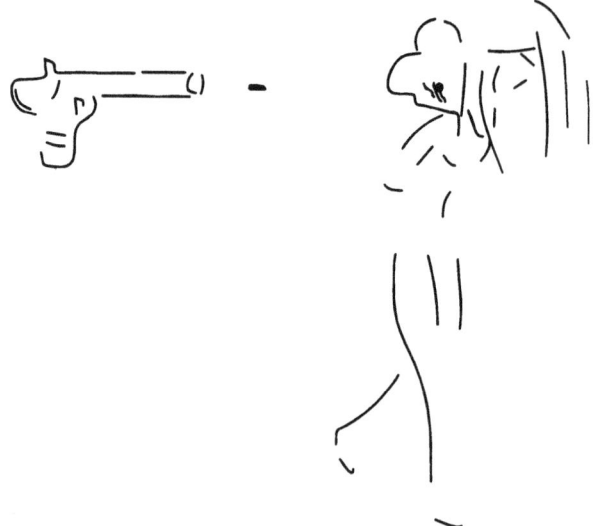

silk on ice

He shows

the only love

he knows

without mercy

His proximity

twists my fears

is he riddled

with cursed intentions?

will my fate

be the same as my past?

trust crushed

again

and again

— hidden agendas

Eyes of kindness
hands of care,
he acted well
to conceal his secret

the dream
he had
to cage me near

Mad Maverick
— untamed
thoughts sever my seams,
this unforgiving world
brings me to my knees

I gave compassion
and found you sly,
you dismissed my grace
venturing every lie

depraved words
revealed your truth,
signs concealed

here my crimson
bleeds once more
beneath your bruise

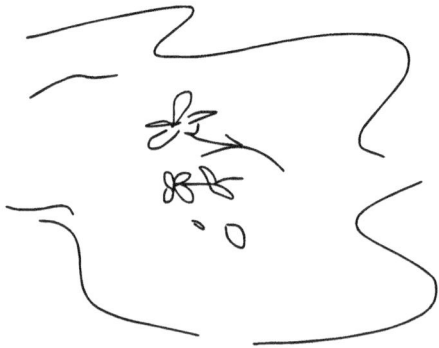

silk on ice

Dealing cards of hearts
I realized I held
his entirety
in one hand

— half a man

He fed silk
on a silver spoon
the kind of words
you'd believe
were nourishing
and full of virtue

but truth be told
he served potions
to hide corrosive lies
a toxic land lived
— masked
behind his broken smile

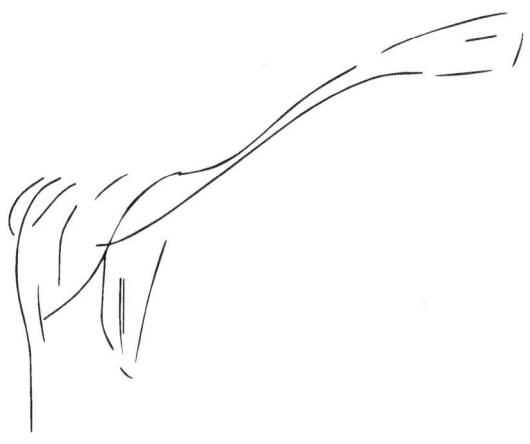

I could sense it
like a hot blade
melting skin to bones

he embedded demons
his joyride —
my unveiling
of his evil descent

paralyzed in fear
a playground in hell
he smiled
and kept his dark secrets
for close friends

too late to escape
a reality
I did not want to hold
too late to protect
the fallen ruins
of a home

Novocaine
you hopeless love
submerging them
beneath the ice,
your freezing
never brings an end
to the wild fires
fear has burned inside

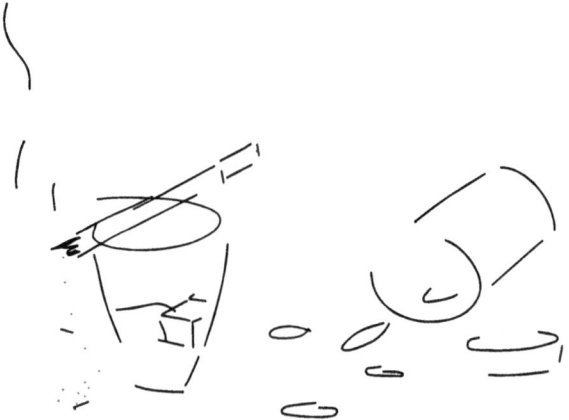

silk on ice

In light

we learn how to love

in darkness

we learn how to run

He wakes —
only to watch me
like prey from afar

— jealousy

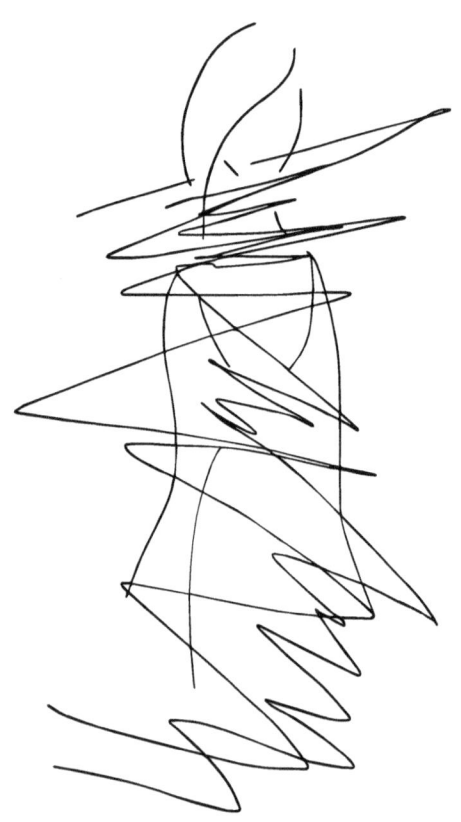

Words hibernate
on the walls I framed,
running through my heart
like open rain

you are my blessing
and the curse
that splits my brain
between discord and sanity

my only inclination
is you are a thief
of my mind

He writes plays
and tells white lies

and on this night
I meet dishonesty
between my thighs

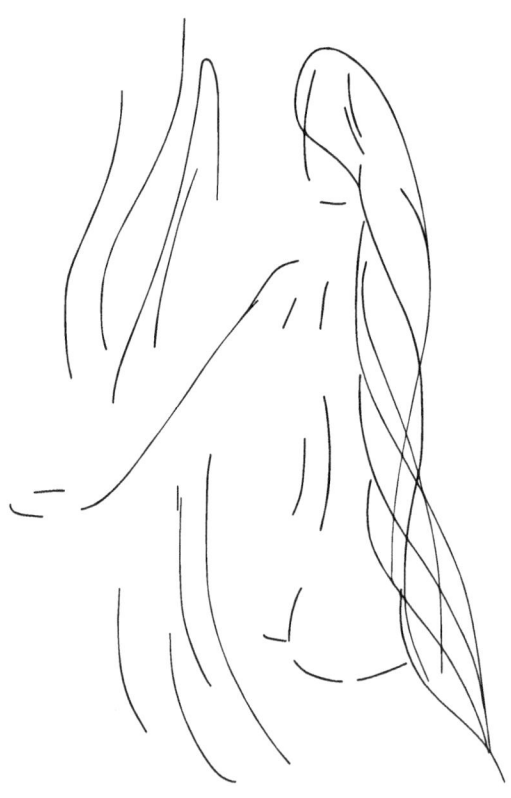

Hail on fire
unleashed a blaze,
thorns pierced my flesh
in a trickster's maze,
he took this body
and cursed my veins

— lying down like
silk on ice
my lips turned blue
knowing *she* did not
deserve the price of
patriarchy's fool

cuts ran deep
between those sheets,
frozen dead
he slayed a queen
and took home bread

Whiskey sour
drips from his lips

every word he speaks
registers rage

— a free spirit
spoiled by anchored chains

casting fish hooks
on an angel's wrist
is a vain heart's game

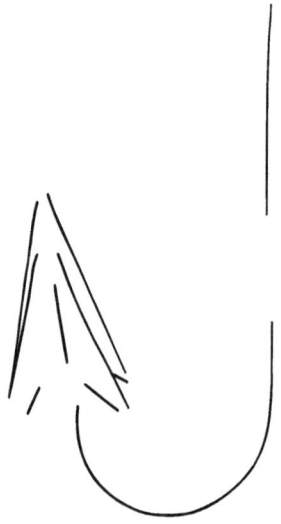

silk on ice

A guy
who licks clit
and talks
is no king of mine

just a generic version
of cheap wine

— players

Blue ribbon
bleeds pink dry,
boys will be boys,
the world exclaims
as truth

this is simply
another excuse

— foul play

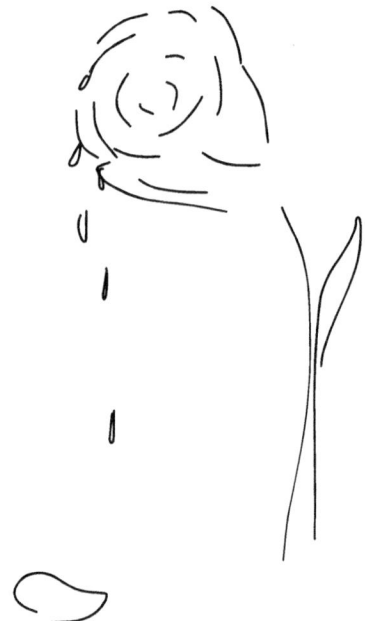

I forgive you, yes
I forgive you, no
I forgive your torment,
I forgive your broken soul

to forgive you
is to forget you,
this one is for you

the give
you get

— karma

Gender inequality,
power and pain,
under this roof it
comes down like rain

why do we yell ...
when we are in this together?

— domestic disputes
reveal world issues

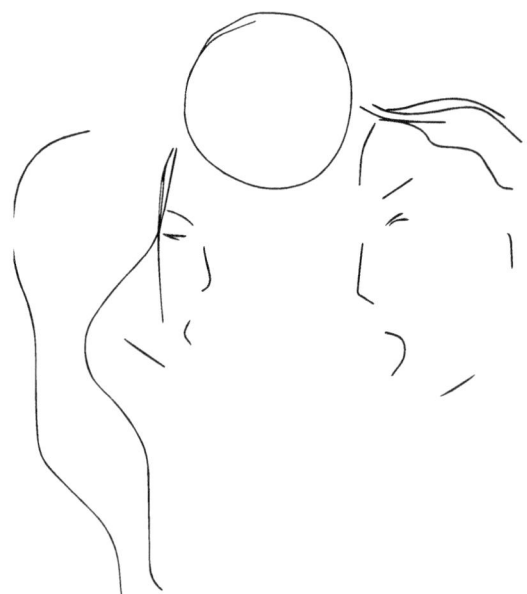

Devoured
by blades of words,
split in two,
it was here
I felt impending doom

he led me into flames
where the furnace brewed
but I knew
words would not burn me
the whole way through

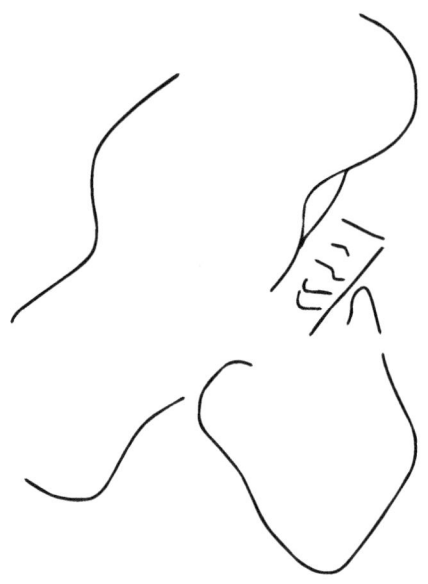

I do not know

what feels cheaper

being laid and left

or

loved and left

they both leave you empty

feeling hurt at the core

He poured me another,
I drank poison,
milky nights
distorted mirrors

I felt the cold beneath me
my fate releasing,
my vessel stale
in ruins and remains
from a tyrant spore
attempting to destroy
my fertile soil

there I stood,
quilting grace
and stitching wounds
with no anesthesia
to ease me through,
intolerable cruelty
I prayed —
love, curb my *cravings* for rage

in the hurricane wave
the *abyss* of me turned mute
there was no mercy,
except to choose
love over fear
the only answer
drenched in truth
— yield to darkness
and you will live through
anything

sian flanagan

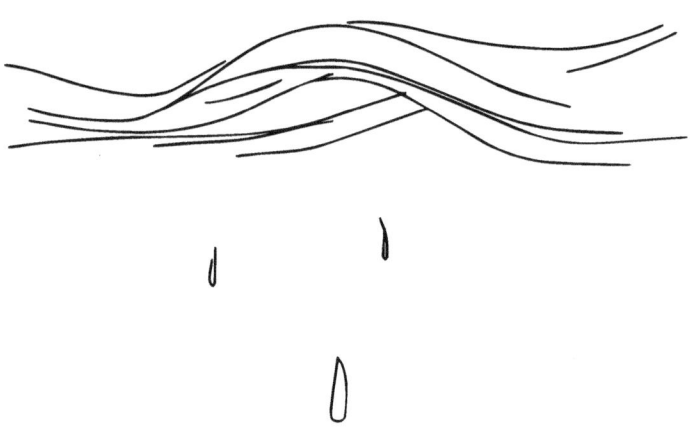

All we do is soak

each other up

to wring each other out

like dirty rags

— battle drops

56

Him versus me
the battle fields merge

a bloodbath of words
shed and spilt

behind closed doors
words bury us
in everything but love

We built a home
on water with bricks
made out of clay ...

sandcastles always crumble
when tides wash away

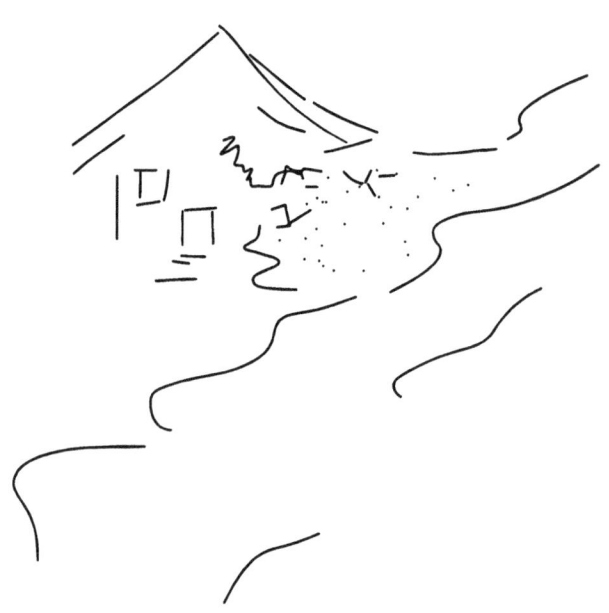

silk on ice

Stargazed

trapped in another

heart's haze

falling

through spells,

lost in a daze

running wild and afraid

He asked: why won't you pour your
heart out into my hands?

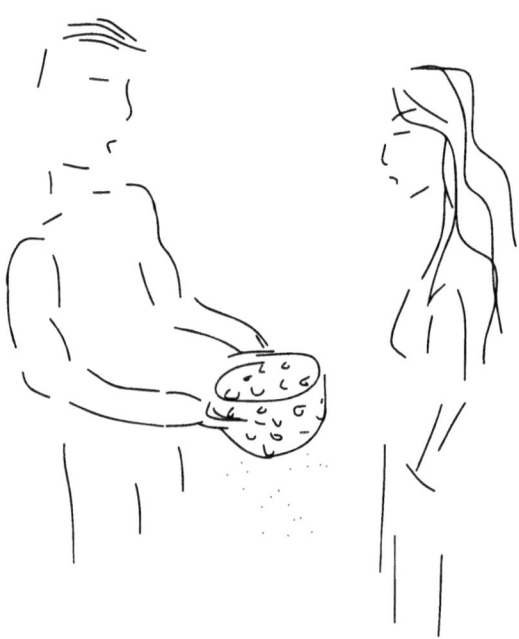

silk on ice

Words boiled over me,
sifting out substance
I learned real taste
by leaving waste
for the drain

Hollow one

caverns deep

words echo

when I speak,

all I hear is a ricochet

of my voice,

my footsteps,

lost in a deserted town,

walking through empty roads

in his lonely land

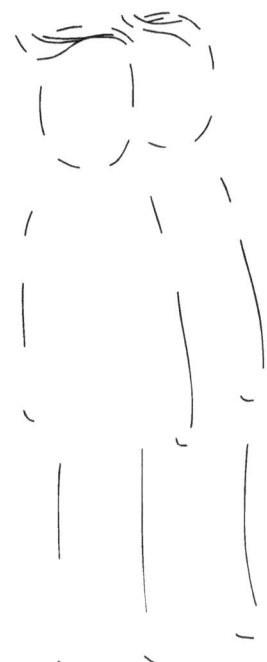

silk on ice

These demons
disturb my sleep,
I lie — restless
contemplating sinful secrets
with dark walls,
justifying all
my battle scars

There is only so many times
we can be pushed and pulled
before we start to shake

— worry

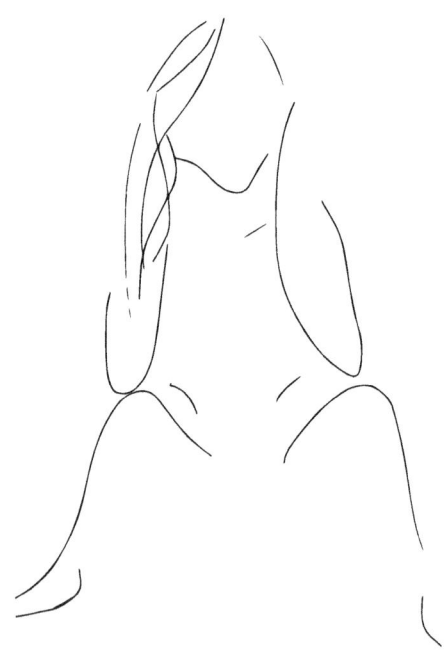

silk on ice

I learned of emptiness
settling for you

— fear

They said:
button up your shirt
tie back your hair
buckle your belt
pull up your socks

stand tall
be strong,
they never said,
this is how
we will learn to wear
our emotions

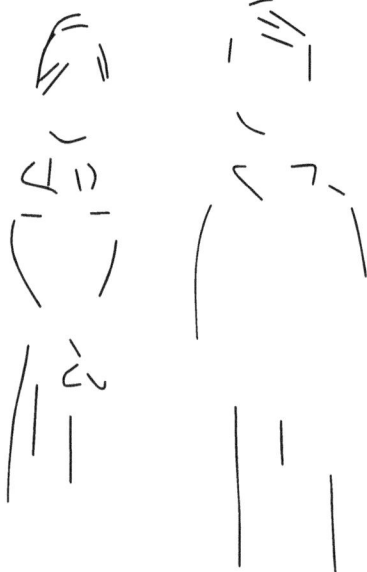

silk on ice

Abandoned
confused
emotionally abused,
this is what it feels like
to be used

— torture chambers

Is my fate warranted

from the form

between my thighs?

— woman

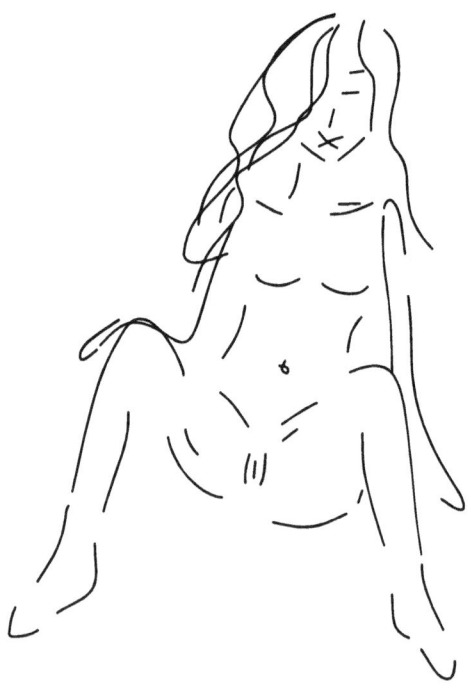

silk on ice

The world acts
like my body
is a board game
for men to play on

this culture of disdain
perpetuates
gender bias games

Silence

will become

your nature

— oppression

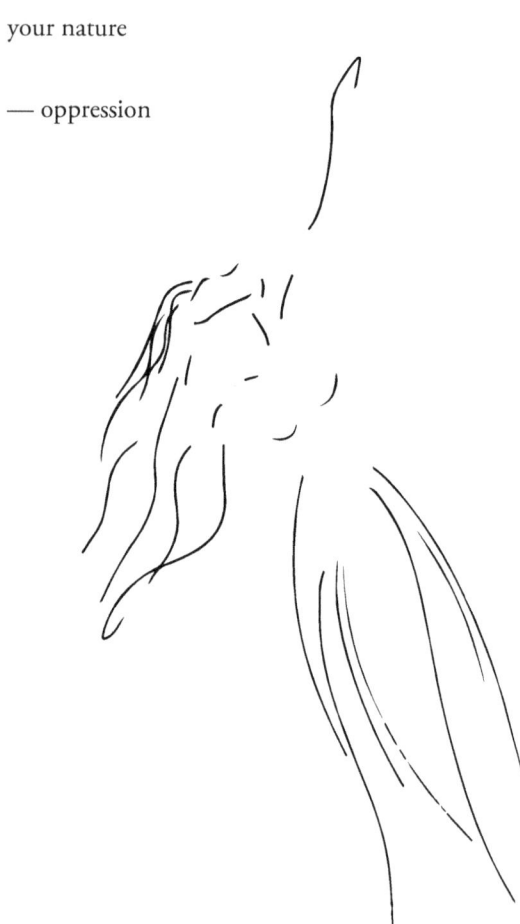

silk on ice

Slut

        Player

she is shamed

        he is deemed a king

double standards
are society's
running game

What is viewed
as forbidden
by culture and men

is a body
a home a place
to sculpt life
and breathe love

a woman's right

— primitive minds

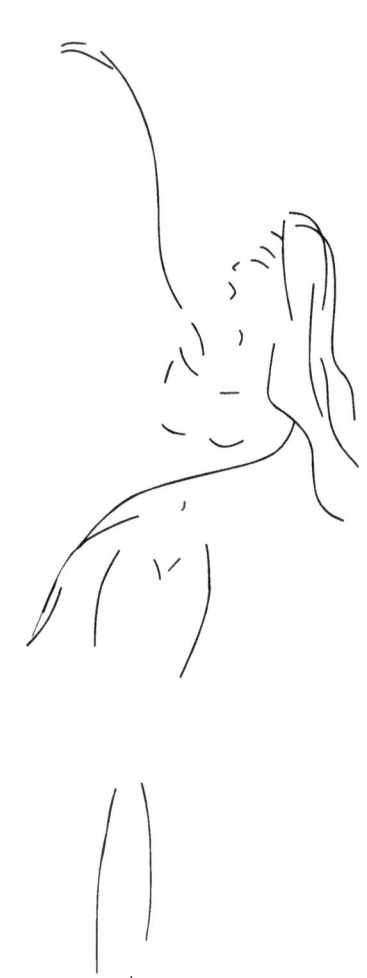

I used to stack my trophies
high up on my shelf

growing up
I came to learn
this is how
some men
collect women

Curvy swerve,

straight and narrow,

skinny mini,

this world plays shallow games,

never a podium

to place or win

just cats being chased by dogs

— society's disorders

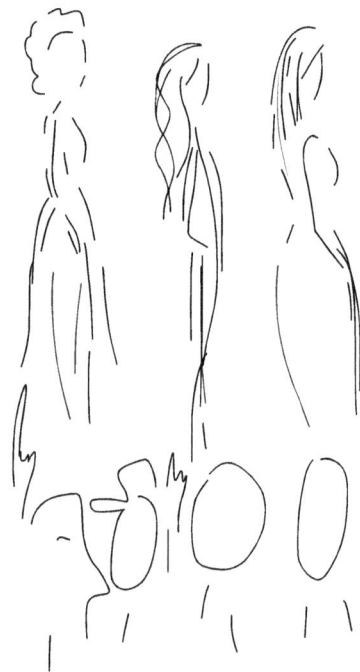

Enculturation breeds
a pleasing personality

— history to present

Be pleasant
talk sweet,
silent opinions
follow pretty's lead ...

how can they expect her
to stand,
when they teach her
how to put bows in her hair
instead of how to grow a backbone?

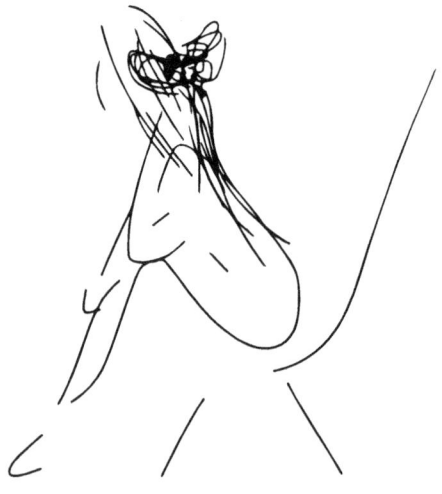

Ladylike ...

does this mean place myself

on the back burner for life?

give up my voice?

be a pleaser?

be easy?

what does it mean to be ladylike?

to do as you're told?

here to be seen and not to be heard?

what does it mean to be a girl?

to play with a doll,

idolizing an unrealistic body shape and size?

to learn that my purpose in life

is to be somebody's wife?

what does it mean to be a woman?

to cater my every move to everyone else,

only to place myself on a dusty old shelf?

how can we

redefine what femininity means

when society keeps telling us

the version we *should* be?

Her eyes stole my soul
with innocence

I wept for her
knowing the world *she* will walk

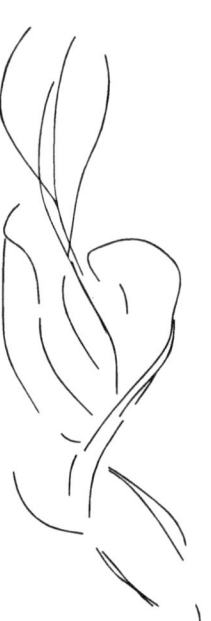

in sorrow
I held her,
leaving tears
in the hands of time

as I gripped her satin skin
between mine

I could not deny the truth
staring into her eyes
— that only knows love

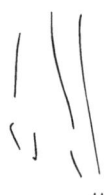

Mother, mother
is it here you feel
lost,
found,
or abandoned?

as your young nestle
into enchanted dreams
— is it here between
nursery rhymes and heartbeats
you pray for girls
to be raised
equal in this world?

for it is here
upon the first beat
of her heart
that she is exiled
from her rightful place,
to stand equal
eye to eye
with all mankind

Inception

the awakening

If you took an oath of silence

the time is now

to reinstate your power

— renegade

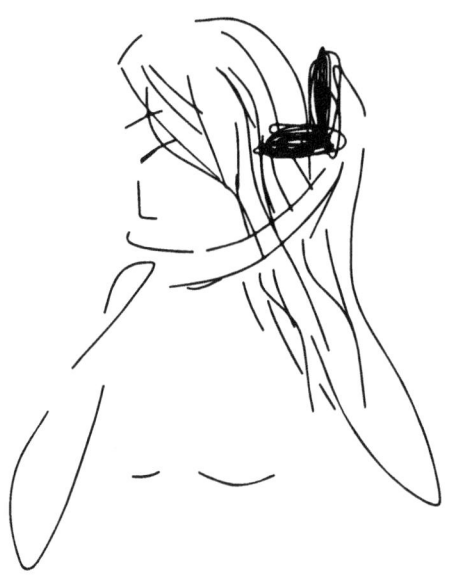

Vulnerability is revered
and yet feared,
here we stand tempted
to reveal and come undone
yet remain riddled,
shaking with anxiety
as we doubt our rightful place
to simply *be*,
and then we wonder
why we cannot be happy

Plunging before the drought

— annihilation

succumbing,

surrendering

this is

resurrection

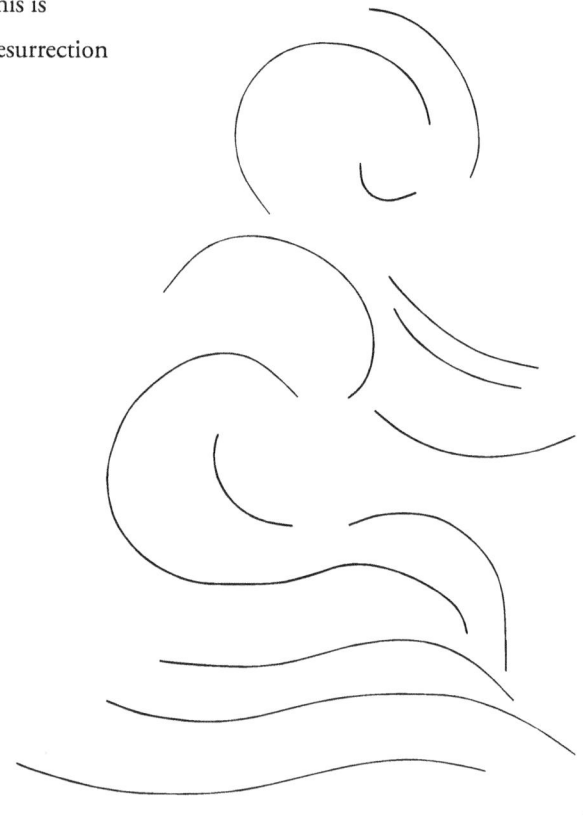

The beat that crowns life
is found
in her eyes
in her arms
beneath her flesh
within her heart

she bared life without requests,
in her hands
she brought you home

this is the mother
the woman
the girl
the goddess
that holds the land of life

the gift —
he has been foolish
to exploit, objectify
and abuse
the home that gave *him*
every reason to love

Love does not
torture this world
conditions do

— conditional love

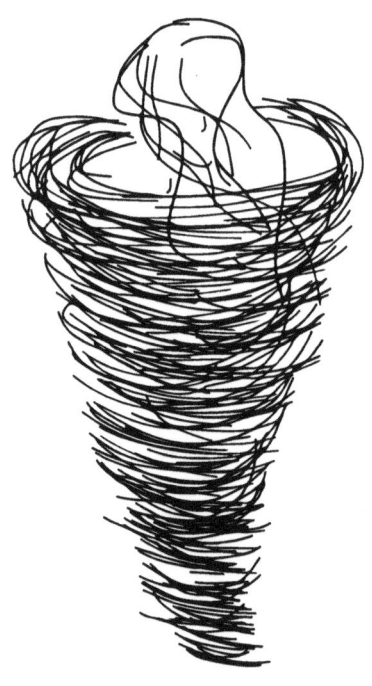

Uterus

the house that carries life,

somehow that justified

the greatest oppression

ever devised by humankind

His frost clothed me
— silence came
the death of us
slowly decayed

love hibernated
as I yearned for spring,
learning to let go
of the frozen world
I used to know

amongst the sleepless cold
my body rested numb

as I surrendered
to renew my form
— marinating love
beneath the storm

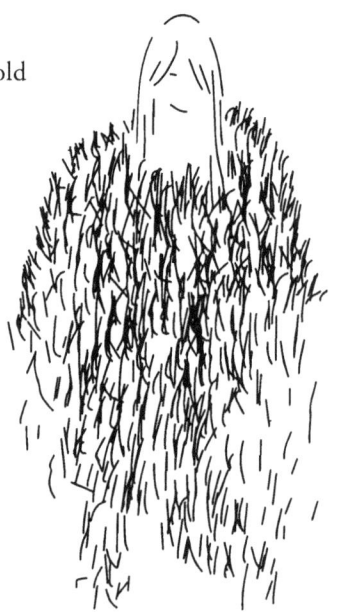

Torn silk
this dagger strips me
piece by piece

he made it his business
to split me in half
— vengeance
is not my act,
healing is all
I ask ...

unfolding,
becoming,
is the only language
I choose to speak

good riddance to the one
who finds pleasure
taking mats out
from underneath
a woman's feet

Scoreboards of war
still exist,
a wise woman told me
tallying games
is a myth
— nobody wins

at the end of days
when washing is done,
under starlight nights
beneath the moon and sun,
the sum of one's existence
surpasses all fights,
somehow we fail to see this
all of our lives

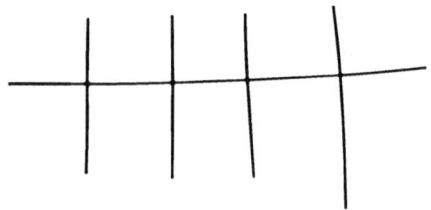

Men think they know best
women often play along
around and around we go
like dogs chasing cars

And there I fell
wings to earth,
I felt a thousand bruises
 from life throwing stones

unjust acts came in waves
rattling these bones,
scar upon scar
I braved this world
with love in my heart
and grace in my hands

now standing tall
as I am
— fierce love
a force that rises
above walls
to answer *the call*

may we all come undone
and rise back home to love

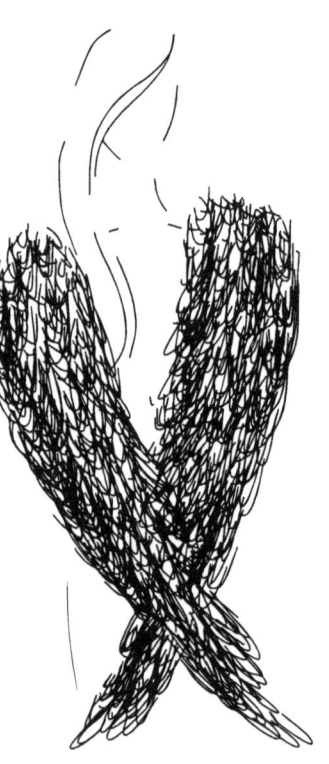

Resurrect with love
cultivate composure,
learn the art of letting go

turn snake bites
into *silk on ice* ...

here,
she found herself
rolling the dice,
rewriting scriptures
beauty once told

there *she* found
a new version
of love to hold

Sometimes
we only know love
when we are caught

in

volatile

ext

r

e

m

e

s

silk on ice

She said: he really loves me though

oh child,
bullets make holes
they don't seal wounds

— defending

Love me

pleaded the child,

remember me

cried the wound

and then I heard my echo ...

love yourself

— *higher self*

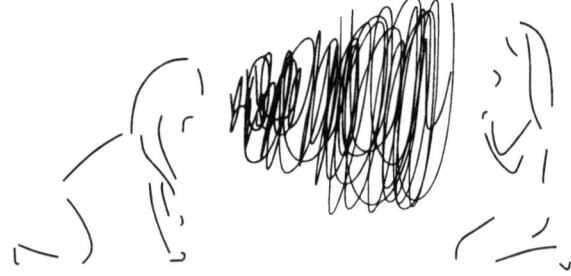

silk on ice

Escaping black holes,
dropping all the words
he told me,
his desires to mold me,
I am not a trophy

letting go,
moving into liberty,
living in my kingdom
this is how I learn to be — *free*

Where did I go wrong?
how did this happen?

oh child —
life is not a path
of happenstance
but rather a course
you carve by hand

thoughts become reality
there is no such thing
as chance

— nature's game

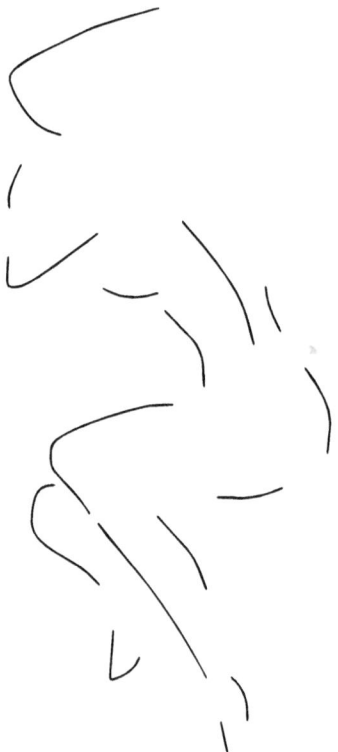

silk on ice

I choose to witness words

instead of hanging

from their ropes

— growth

Tell me ... how do I vanish these thoughts?

— unplug

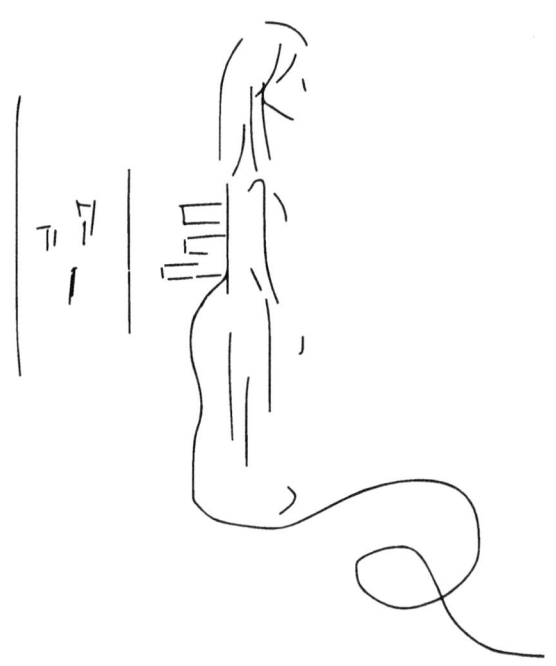

Infractions toward
the *self*
manipulate reality,
fractures split bones
into brittle leaves,
both bring agony

corruption of thought
leads an army of villains
into one's sacred nest,
as ill thoughts compete
to leave their legacy,
siphoning out one's best

Rip this jagged
edge of vanity
from the flesh
that keeps me warm

— ego

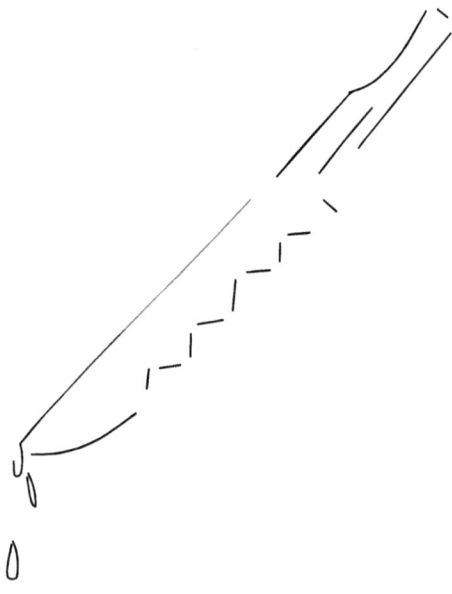

silk on ice

Painting faces
for the masquerade
from sunrise to sunset
day after day ...

how much time do we spend
decorating our bodies
versus loving ourselves?

Repression of self
restrains the authentic
essence inside

challenges offer us the journey
of relearning how to climb

stretch yourself
to reign in your light,
reframe
your inner mirror
with pure delight

Clinging on
this ego steers me wrong

confused,
afraid,
rage buried
beneath the hurt

this matrix evil
has me conjuring fake suits

driving wild
she takes the wheel,
she's on the loose

setting fire to rain
she blazes away

— shadow play

Have I lost my edge?
am I becoming less of who I am?

no child —
remember,
square pegs do not fit
into round holes

we lose our edges
so we become whole

— coming undone

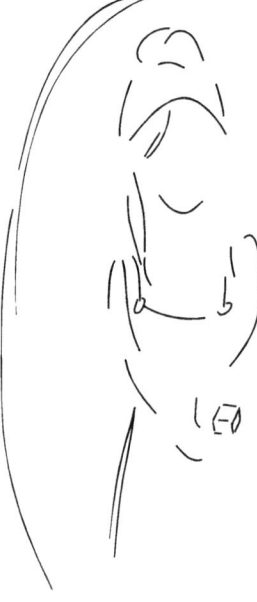

silk on ice

Caught in the wrath
of indignation?
— good
stay there
until you are fed up
with negativity,
then turn the page
and start again

Sometimes you have to break

your own heart

to know what love is …

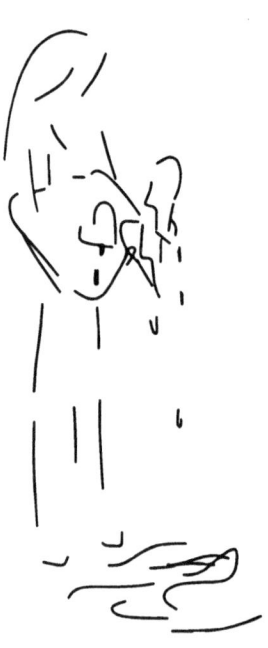

Careful —

this ego thing

will make you porous,

so much so

when another gives

you will not

know how to receive

and there,

you will stand holding nothing

but an empty vessel

— alone

wondering why

no one is willing

to settle for your crumbs

Too skinny

too fat

too thin

too thick

remember when we did not

torment ourselves

with foolish thinking?

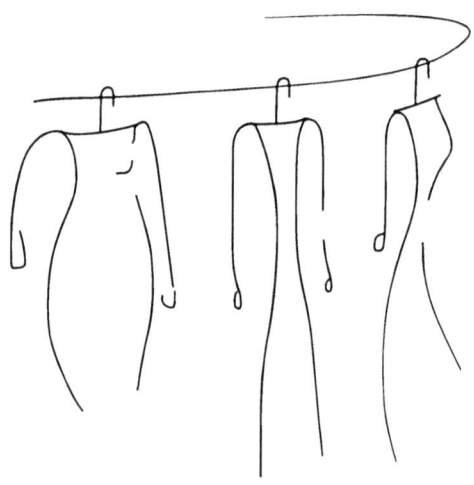

silk on ice

Comparison
plays cat and mouse,
a never-ending war

judgment,
jealousy,
the cause of segregation

we were too young
to know words cut like knives,
too insecure to care
we were building a tyranny
that could stand the test of time

— catfight

When numbing
becomes a safe haven,
feelings,
sensations,
get lost
— a relief not to feel
when you have felt so much

but numbness drinks the youth
from livelihood,
reality fades
you risk too much
— to feel is to know
you are alive

— revive

Funny how
we collect things
in attempt to
hold and keep,
we take away our freedom
by claiming nouns
with more attachment
than our dreams

— grasping at things to keep
becoming prisoners
to our pleasures

a culture built on false illusions
worshipping external treasure

this is the culprit
of the Western world's addictions

Let it drain out
wash away cells of
clutter,
stress,
resentment and hate,
run your canvas
through a hot bath,
submerge,
rinse off the dirt,
shed layers that do not serve,
release the hurt,
find the beat of your drum,
believe in stars and
a good heart once more

— let go

Growing into love
— nothing feels eternal
but drinking her wine

I said,
there is no reason
for me to bring my life to you
other than to lose it,
I just want to know you
and then disappear

she whispered,
knowing me
does not mean dying
my dear

— surrender

Life is a vortex,
a jungle,
full of wickedness
and beauty

a master plan
illuminating
perfection in paradox,
like a rose held
by a stem of thorns

finding one's way
through thick brush
will be an adventure
or a nightmare

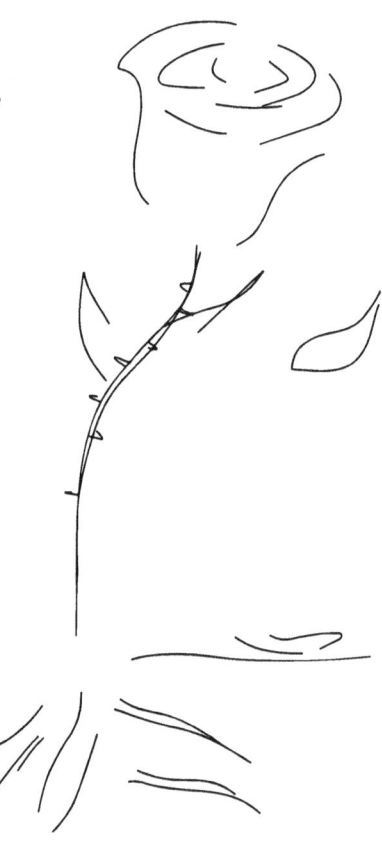

silk on ice

The older I get
the more I realize
the seeds of truth
rest in every child,
that everything here
is on borrowed time

and nothing
we have we will ever keep,
there is now
and now,
this is
what matters most

so for the love of life,
free yourself
from history's ghosts

And then she left
fields that wilted her soul

no longer
stricken to barren lands
that made her cold

she ran
to the world she had always known
— amongst intrepid horizons
her wonderland arose

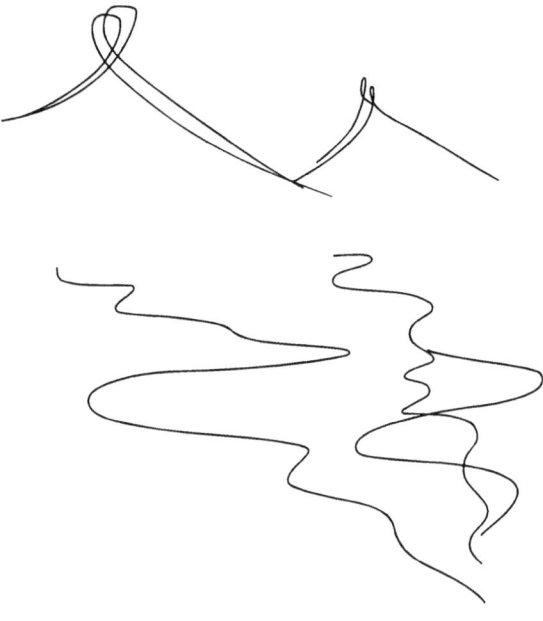

Feel,

emerge,

unzip the dungeon

that only knew of hurt,

slip through the cracks

of night's hands

illuminate,

be seen,

rise to earth,

open your eyes

you are alive

young girl

— rising

I slipped down somberly
I felt rain upon me
with every drop
I heard each note

I listened,
feeling forgiveness
wash over my heart
healing the curse,
and there
I found my way
through words
told by rain

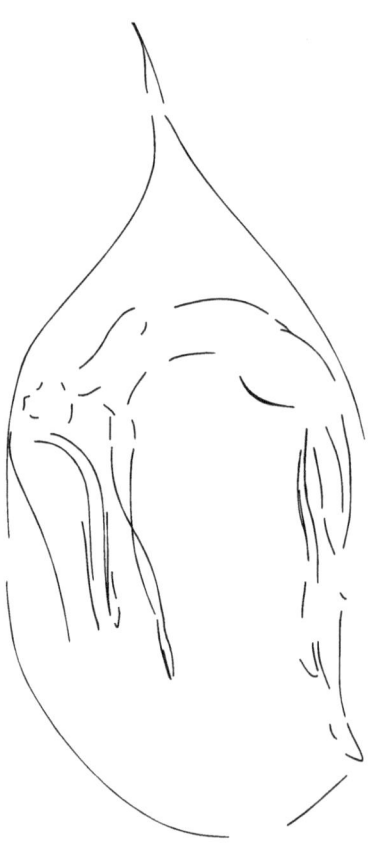

leaving the
fractures
of blame,
pointing toward
the future
knowing scars
are not for fame,
but rather,
love for thy self
is the vibrant way

If we care to watch
we can find
beauty and meaning
in between
the drips and drops
of life

Intuition protects you

ego conflicts you

— truth versus lies

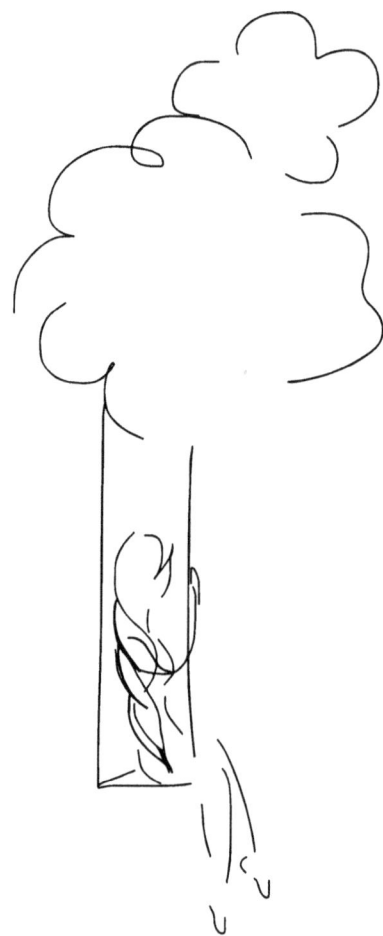

silk on ice

If I live cautiously
I will die of a broken heart,
for I am cursed and blessed
to seek adventure toward the stars

so here — I live
jumping cloud to cloud,
a skywalker,
riding every wave of thunder
that tries to strike me down

here — I fly
living up and away
without the laws of gravity
to save me from this place

may my heart grace me
with strength
to seize this day

Forget the past

it is not your future,

you decide

where your journey rides

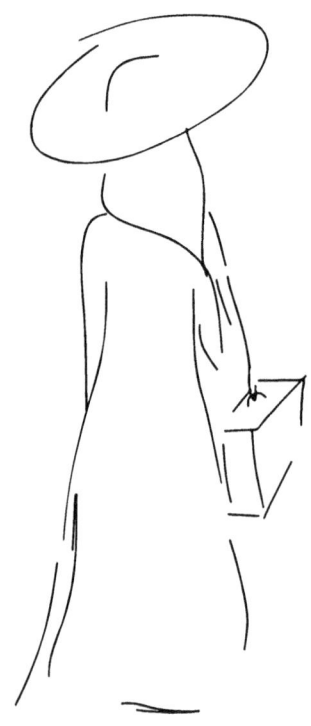

I dare you to leave
the fallacies
and face the truth
awaken the eclipse
that reveals real fruit ...

awaken
from the shadow
that keeps you drinking
the bitter taste of sour

surrender
what does not serve
your world,
unlock your innate power

choose with dignity
to dress and rehearse
the callings
that ignite the best of you

Love
feeling grace

Falling in love
is a gift,
a privilege,
a unicorn
few are fortunate
enough to meet

like the tales and mysteries
of mermaids beneath the sea

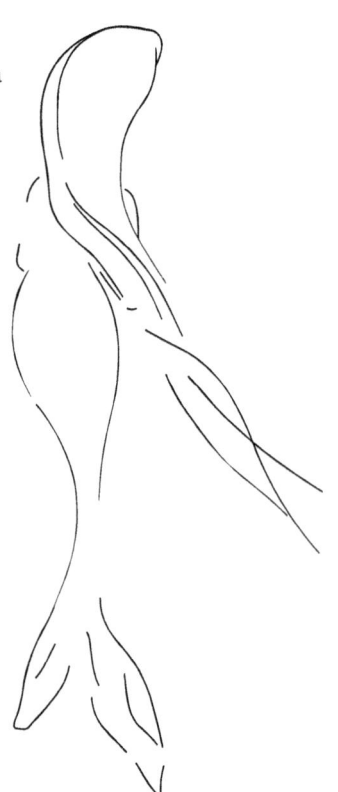

silk on ice

Love lives
in hearts that see
rainbow-colored snow,
even through thick ice
love carves silk paths
to bring you home

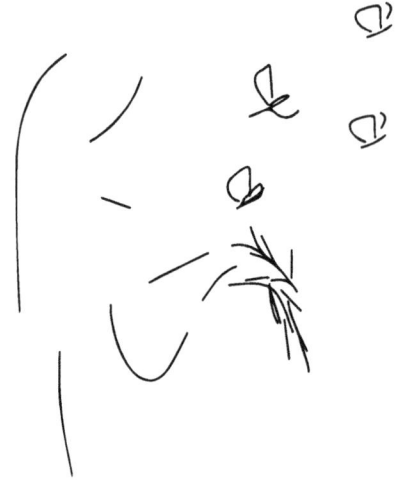

My landscapes
are full of adventure
come away with me
into uncharted terrain

let's be like butterflies
learning of their wings
again
for the first time

Your presence is adored
and desired like lemonade

you are the energy
that sweetens
the juice of my life

It is from this love
I know why people
do not want
to grow old

— playing for keeps

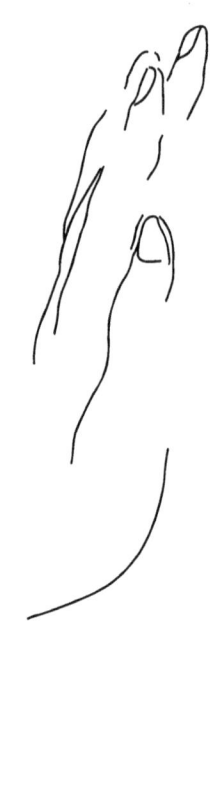

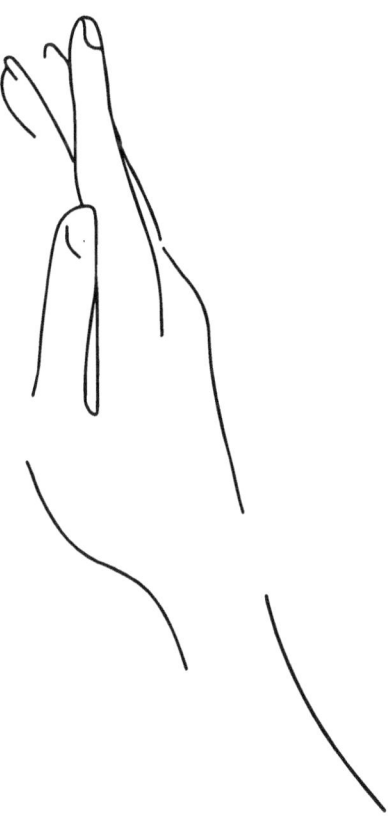

While the world sleeps
and pillows perform their duty
resting bedheads and beauties,
come away with me
to the moon and back

He said:
I want to chase
the world with you
come!
let's catch night rides,
let's whisper words on
midnight trains
and fire shooting stars
in the dark
till dawn awakens

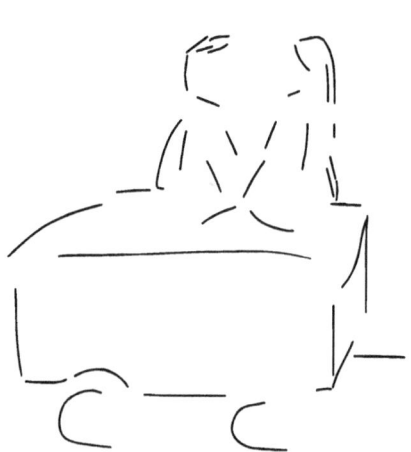

silk on ice

Playful
witty
charming
cute

this song
in my stereo
reminds me of you

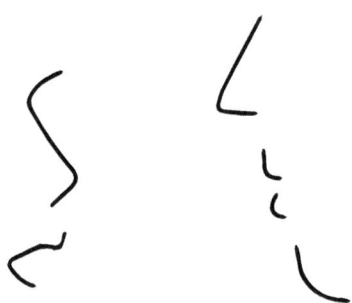

You are the mirror

reflecting

the world

within me

— relationship

You are the meadow
in my dark,
a sweet embrace
when the world turns gray

your essence holds
still waters clear
overseeing
life's nebulous games,
chivalry still runs
through your veins

you are my wonderland
weathering all storms,
through the sands of time
— the heart I call home

you are —
my whisper
my cathedral
my steed of love
my soul's ever after
in this lifetime and those to come

— one and only

Moments dissolving
fleeing the hands of time

but this one here
I will cherish
for a thousand moons

— with you

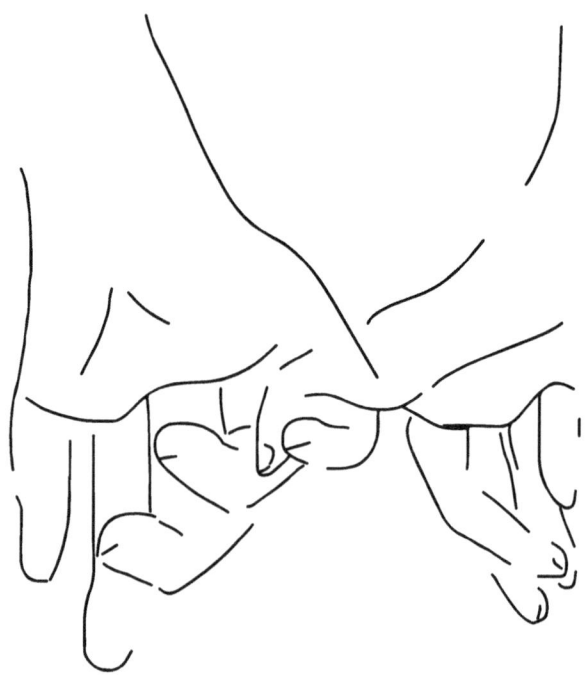

Twisting and turning
on empty roads,
unraveling
weathered vines wrapped
in the biography of my soul

it is only through resting
on the wings of memories
I once called home
that I am fuelled to carry on

my heart seeks
the pulse of his touch,
for it is him
that presses me
to live into eternity

so I can find him again
and again
and again
always and forever

What whispers feel like

in the dark

next to you

— love bombs

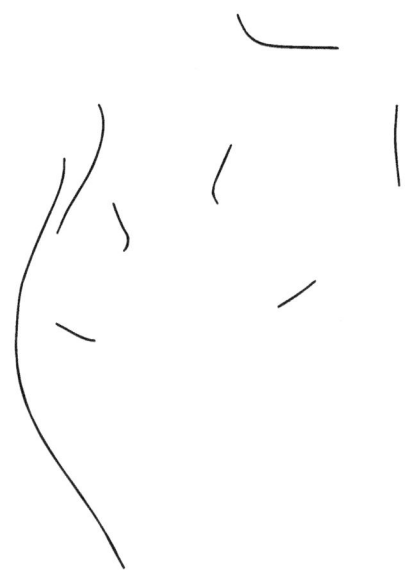

silk on ice

Vanilla rooibos

cream to my lips

smooth to the touch

you taste

like wildflowers

born in spring

the kind of love

I only want to

breathe in

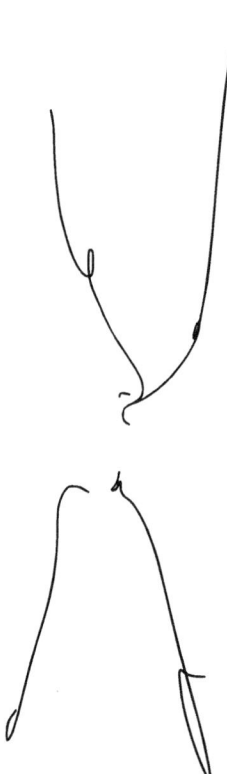

Lips meet —
my gut knows
I'd rather be alone
than feel nothing
at all

All or nothing
impavid for you
twisted in your beauty
too good to be true

broken past
leaning through the aftermath
stumbling upon utopia,
all eyes on you

rolling on through
fearless for you

He tastes like poetry
bringing me to my knees,
I feel like *silk* at the mercy
of his squeeze,
his touch grips my innocence
and I enjoy
every minute of it

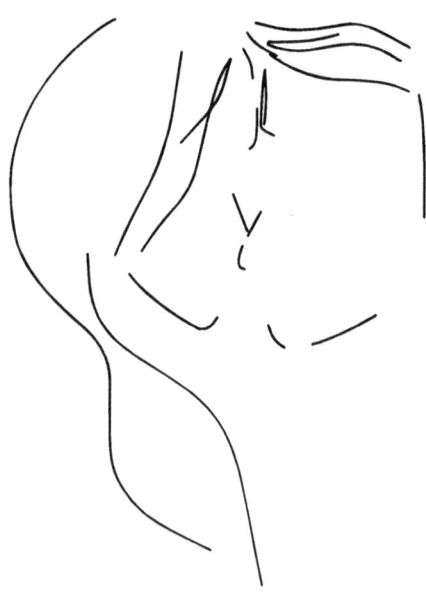

silk on ice

I would give you the world
but then
I will forever be at your mercy

— love spell

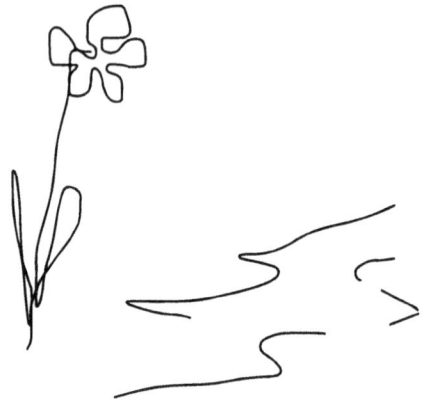

I stumbled onto your banks,
I sat peacefully
watching you flow
learning of your soul

when I saw you
for the first time
and knew
I was *home*

silk on ice

I wonder —
how many times I have searched myself
only to unearth the seed that yields
your calling

I wonder —
how many moons and galaxies
I have sought, in time,
knowing, I would find you
and all this love
would be won and lost once more

again and again
our memories are slain
into white ash
where sand meets the shore

only to find you once more,
bid you hello,
I love you
goodbye —
for you are my soul's complement
as we play within the mortal plague,
the waiting game of love
lost and found in time

He whispered:
I will never falter
as long as I live beside my queen
for the ocean of her love
encapsulates me

in the purity of her depths
I could be left breathless
and still be full of life

for I hold a goddess
close to me tonight

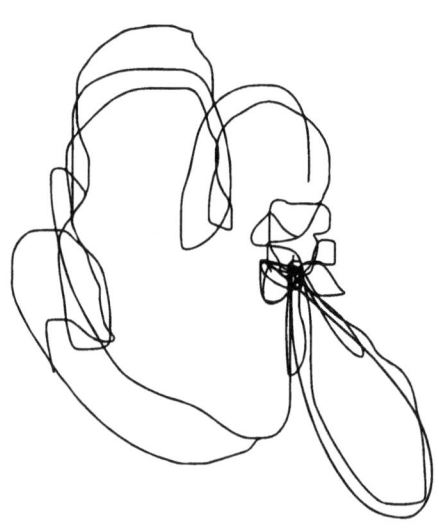

silk on ice

This lay of love
has sealed me completely
for an instant

— orgasm

His fingers unlock me
code after code,
free-falling
between my knees,
naked *silk* paints
us seamlessly

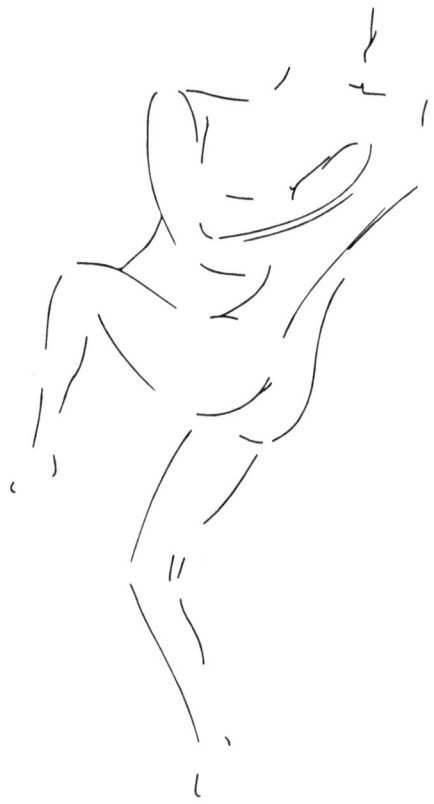

Magician —
he speaks love,
he knows my lips,
he knows my heart,

he knows me as a divine woman
I know him as a divine man

this world
is our world
together we create
our wonderland

— equality

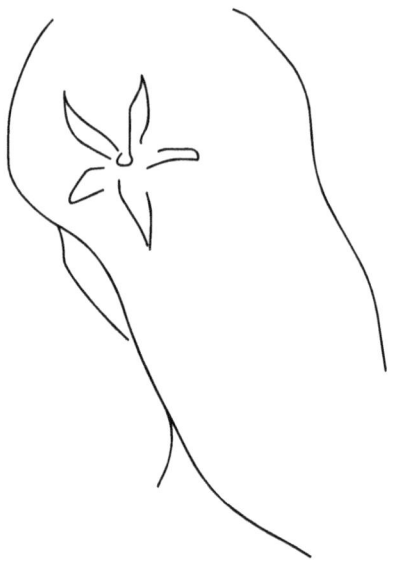

Magic wands

know wizardry

wild dreams

lead me on

— fantasies

69 is a good demonstration

of give and take

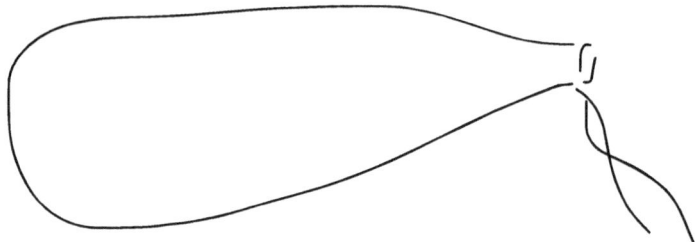

No one stimulates
my appetite like you,
not even red velvet wine

you are the nectar
I long to drink,
the evanescence
I kiss in daydreams,

the abstract paint
layering white,
the song I sing
each night

In a glance
he undresses me

we move
from nightfall till dawn,
let us always be this young

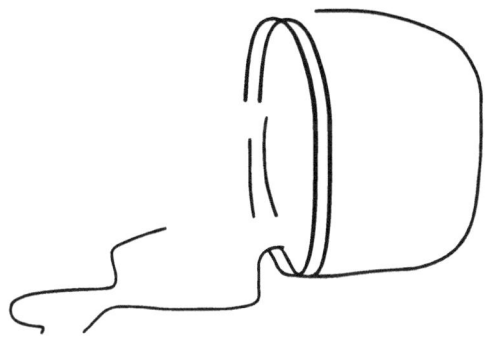

Bend me like clay

unfold me like sunrise

does the day

take me high,

where our spirits play

shape the space

between us,

where words

have no place

where head to toe

our wild souls

moan

I love you
is a fairy tale,
a tragedy,
caught along the spines
of roses and their thorns

— a paradox
born between heart and mind,
fluency and discord,
an evergreen,
an island
lost and found at sea
a mesmerizing oasis,
a fond meme

Love is an enigma of the mind
but a true frequency
of the heart

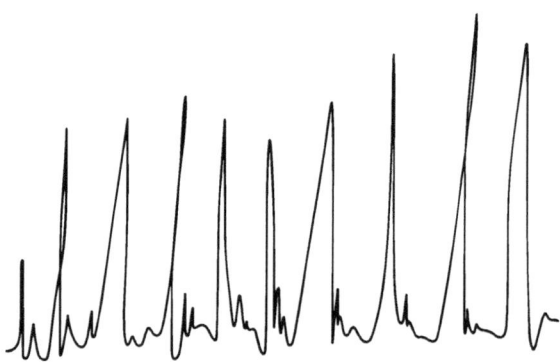

silk on ice

When you fall in love
strap your moon boots on,
plant your feet firmly
on solid ground

grow roots
feel into love

instead of falling
out of your mind

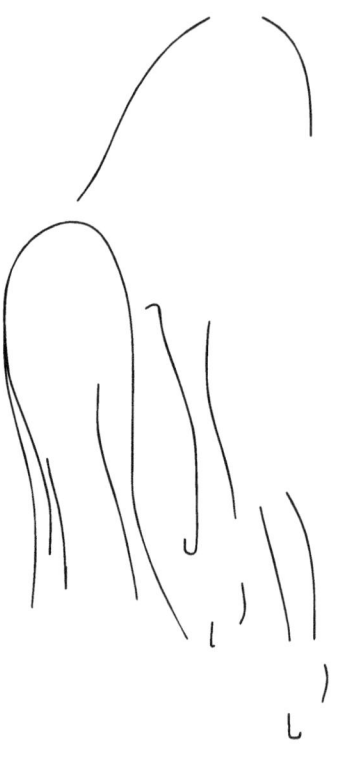

Hand in hand
we walk the line
toward thunder

knowing —
the impending fall
that follows
lightning's strike

these steps reminisce
down memory lane,
hello,
goodbye,
the last dance we know
ends tonight

— lovers born and left

I love you
is not a plan
to have you
nor to hold
or keep

I love you
means
I am here —
unconditionally
so you can discover the parts of you
that could not unfold alone

this is true companionship
— holding space
for you to be whole

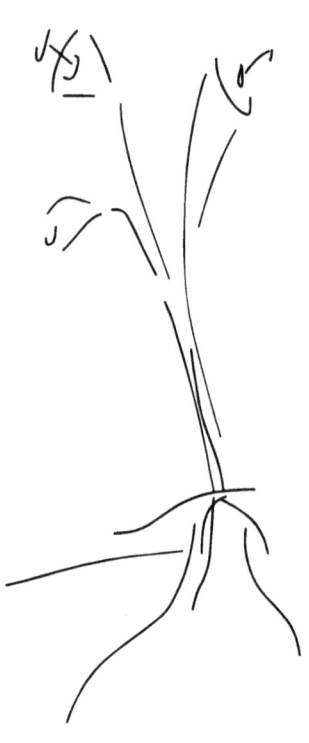

Missing poetry,
I yearn for his vines
to weave intimate roots,

oh, how I wish
for him to come alive
like sunshine in June

may vanity fade
and let the wonderland
I know he holds
unfold with time's rays

Peace —
rain over this world
let your seeds soak
and yield fruit
in those
who wish to drink
and clothe themselves
in your truth

Butter and spaghetti
such a boring dish

that's what he tasted like
plain food
with no spice
not something
I could eat for life

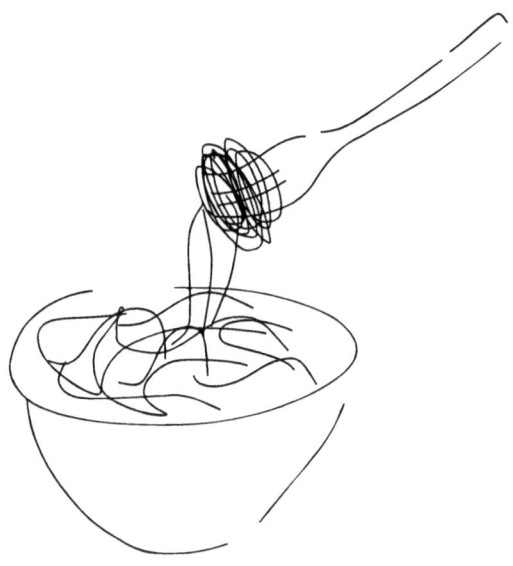

And then anew
came so soon,
I took a walk
in Central Park
with a man I barely knew,
I took a chance —
when he held out his hand
and swore against the tale,
all is fair in love and war
— I took a chance in NYC,
meandering streets,
wandering through the Met
gazing at Monet's best
and all these moments
arrived and left
with one quick flight
and fleeting steps
— dearly departed
there we rest
in memories
cursed and blessed,
full and empty at best,
in the end
love and war
was always fair play

A boy can't hold you
in his hands

choose a man
with hands that can

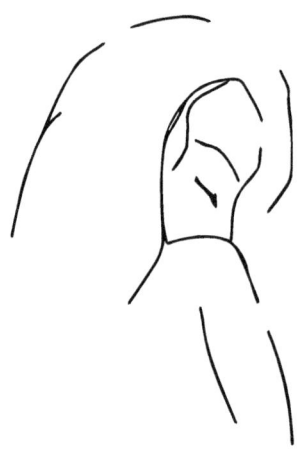

silk on ice

He said:
you are too much

and she replied:
ah yes,
but I am
someone's favorite
late-night kiss
underneath the stars,
I won't be settling
for one who does not know
how to hold so much
in his arms

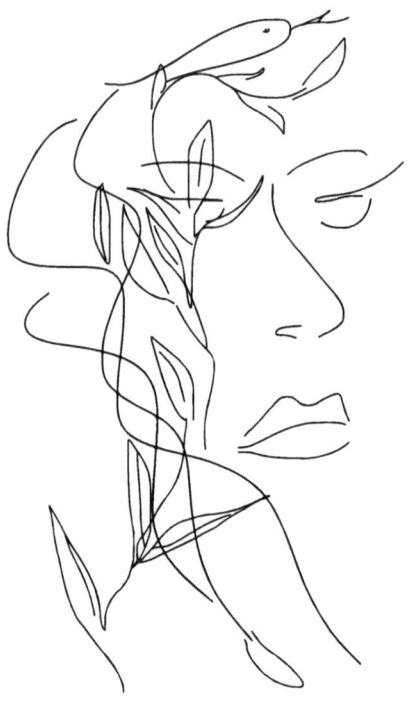

If you want to know

a real man

challenge his beliefs,

see what happens

when he's caught off his feet

are values breached?

does strength hold his honor or

does his truth reveal a coward?

Words lash,

boy —

know playing with dragons

is not a fair game,

you'll get caught in her fire

and beg for rain

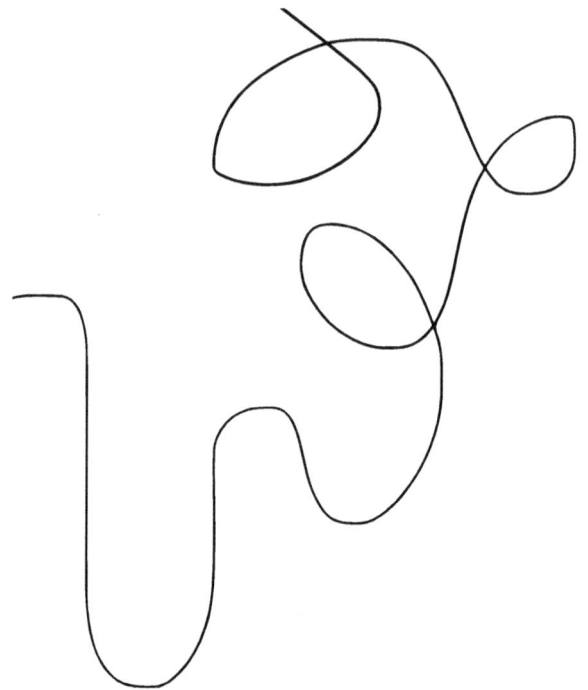

Relationships

are not linear streams

they curve and wobble

like roller coasters

and wild dreams

— enjoy the ride

Love is simple
often sweet
but true love
cares enough to challenge
all your false beliefs,
so you can truly know love
in good company

so forgive me
if my love feels like transgressions
more than affection,
for I mirror blind spots
that cannot be found
in your reflection

too often we rest concealed
beneath our underworld,
held hostage by the lies
we were taught
all of our lives

— recover
what you failed to believe,
love awaits you unconditionally

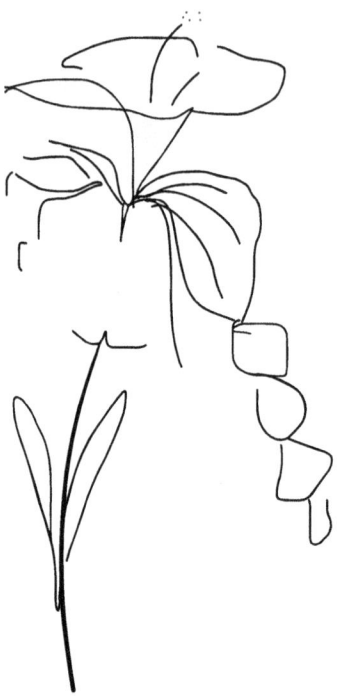

I don't want to be your night
I want to be your sunrise

— commitment

Shy bird
I see your smile

it's the same language
denial tries to hide

I see — you feel guilty
with feet moving so quickly

caught
between the fabric of time,
standing in two worlds apart

you only offer
half of your heart

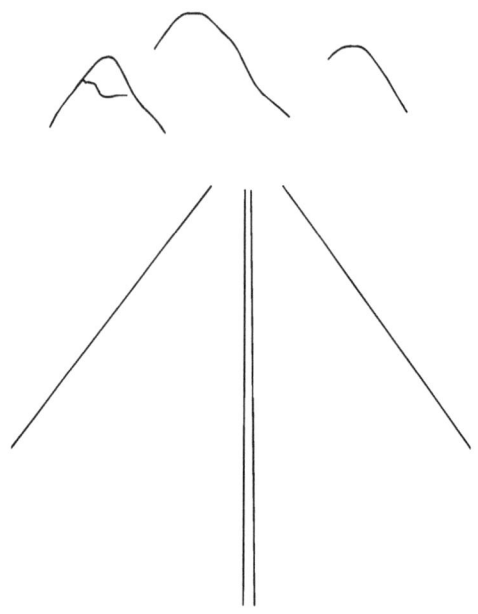

My senses expelled
with your departure

I watched —
as rubber followed highway lines

I held my breath
with the taste of summer rain
and bittersweet goodbyes

Men
lost their use
with genuine words
but you know chivalry
like an ethereal touch

a heart so true
love so deep
real feels
so new to me

I fear
to fall prey
to love
— I long for truth
beyond the wonder
you exude

In serendipity we meet
perfectly imperfect,
flowing with words
and inspiration,

at first bloom
satin petals met sunlight

and now,
we dance our own dance
peering at opposite ends
of the moonlight

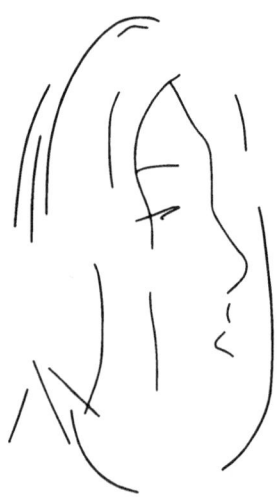

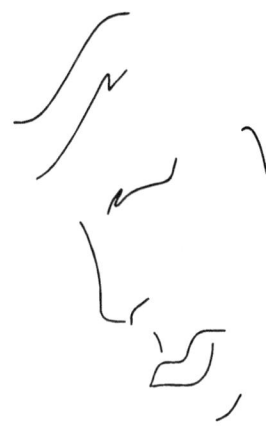

This isn't a love song
but this is our song,
everything that went wrong

You cared too much

he cared too little,

this is how one heart slowly dies

while the other feels

nothing different

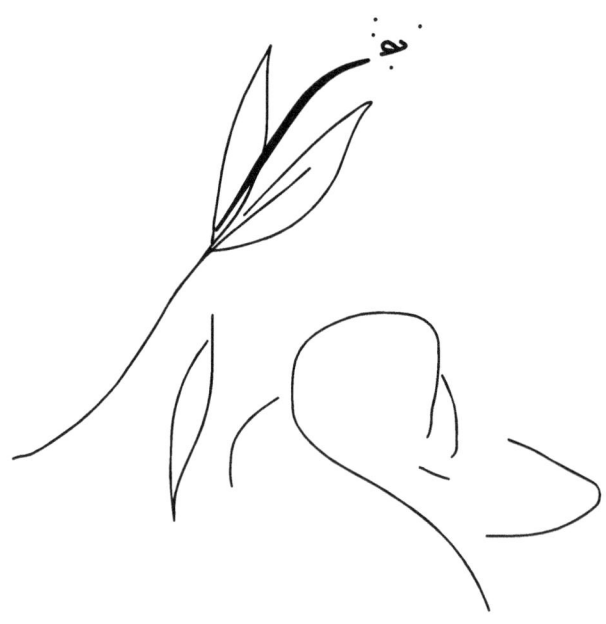

Underneath the stars
when light shines
above us all

I whisper to the moon
I love you
I miss you
good night

— goodbye

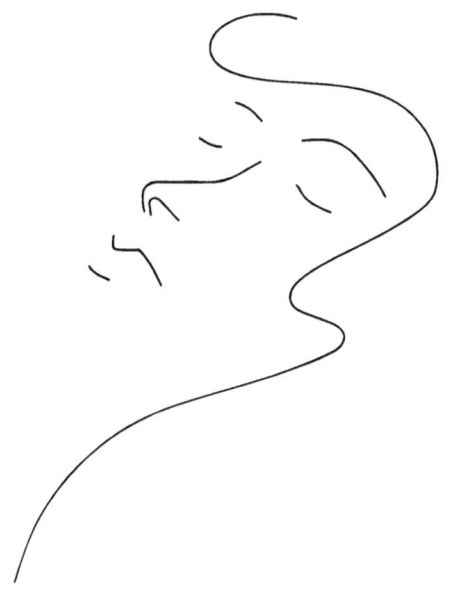

Do we intrigue and engage
each other's minds
or are we here to
pass the time?

— ceiling chatter

Home
a scent of pine,
a calm embrace
in turbulent times,
year after year,
brick after brick,
hand in hand,
what drove us to burn candles
into flames?

love — made from two
and yet we depart from
the same blankets and pillows
we once slept on

the wheelbarrow
stopped turning,
our work — done,
the gardens dug up,
a kiss moved on

dearly beloved
we are gathered here today
saying goodbye to the home we built
and the love we left in pain,
we loved so much
and then walked away,
to evolve,
to be more of who we are
in this life and the next

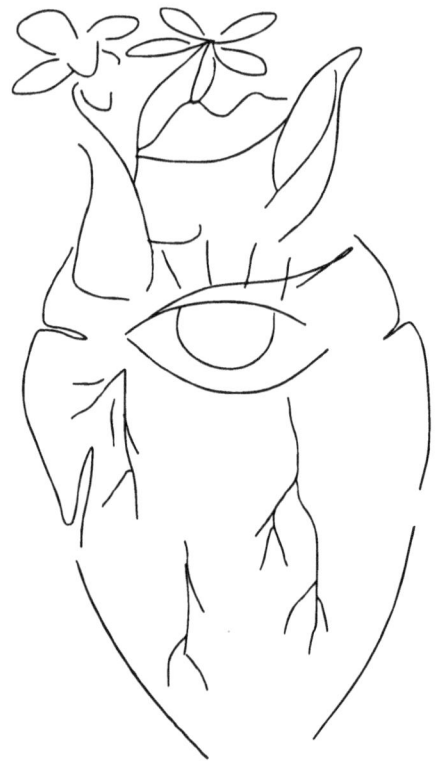

Trust is the secret key

to threading *silk* with your hands,

let intuition bring you

a real man

Love leaves
paper trails,
notes,
letters,
and receipts
full of memories
that taught you — true love
and what it means
— the kind of affection
that makes you want
to carve ink on your arm,
the same warmth you feel
humming your favorite song
— he is the type of man
you pray your daughter meets,
a man who has the strength
to set you free
and still love you
unconditionally,
the one
everyone told you to keep
— he knew love
before you understood it
you held back
even though he wouldn't

Swords and shields

do not give men purpose

hearts do

— love dismisses war and ego

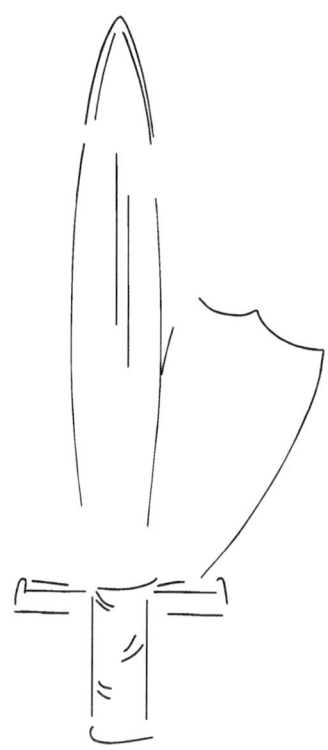

You know the measure of a man
by the length of mercy
he holds in his hands,

you know the persistence of a man
by his willingness
to lead with the word — can

you know the morals of a man
when his gentleness is a pasture
he holds close to his inner land

you know a real man
when his strength shows tears,
when his heart reveals his fears

Show me a boy
who knows all women
are divine mothers of life
and I will show you a *man*

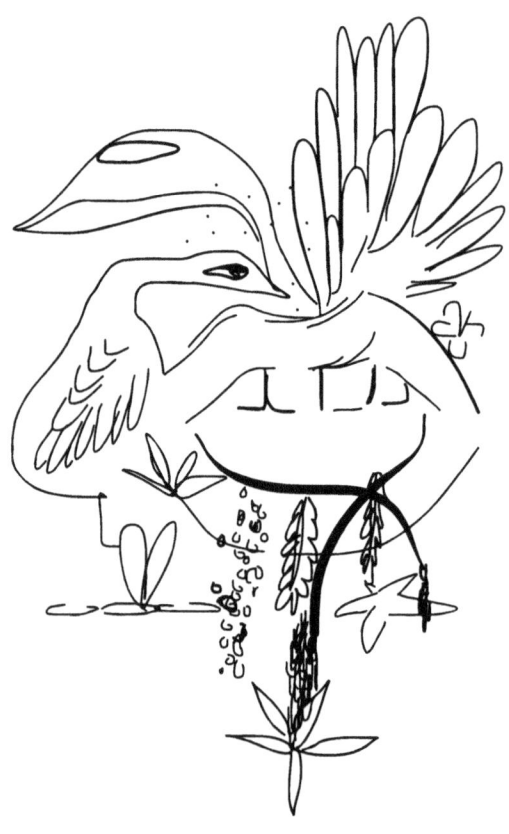

silk on ice

He said:

being with a woman

shows you everything

that matters most,

knowing her is endless,

my respect for her is timeless

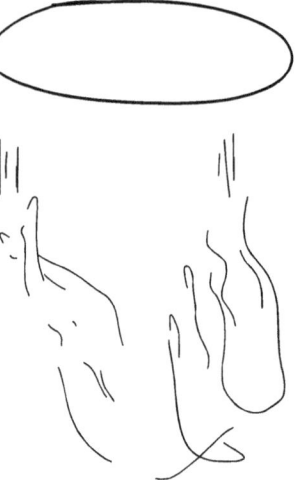

We are so tempted to keep
what could potentially flee
so we worry
and nag
expressing jealousy

but this style of thinking
is our insecurities
grasping at straws,
not realizing
negativity tears down
our internal walls

leaving us empty
instead of full,
this is where
we fall through

The crux of it all
is we can never have
someone or something —
that is the great myth,
the loss
and the hearty heart
of love

in the end
it was always
all or nothing

— borrowed time

There is something so fragile
and innocent about love

something we often forget
trust is easily
won and lost

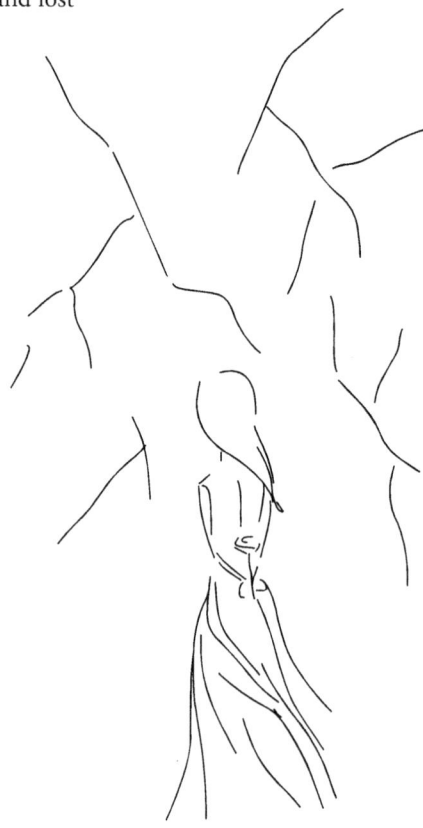

We can count our lucky stars
we are not meant to win
the affection and approval
of many

this leaves room
for truly loving a few
who are ready

The drum of morning
beats through my chest,
this day comes
showering rays for all to reign

and here we stand
with all to hold
and none to keep
except the nectar
we instill and breed

pulse of day
set me on fire,
draw from the passion
that ignites my flare,
lead me on my way,
let grace run through me
on this day

Love does not temper,

jealousy does,

love does not lock doors

it parts the sky,

love always lives

in the rise of morning

and at the end of goodbyes

love is not,

I did and you didn't,

love is not always formal —

but rather embodies

an oxymoron

this is why love

takes strength

because love is simple

yet we make it complex

A face

not a *pretty* place for long

just an image

a shell —

my mind is the stratosphere

where love is made,

where sex feels

like silk sheets

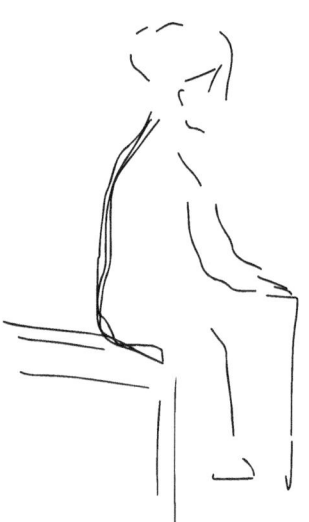

my body is not a sin

it is my home

not a place

for ignorance to roam

my heart is the gravity

that magnetizes one's soul

my celestial

radiates beauty and strength,

the evanescence

a man

aspires to feel

and meet

You

are not your body

your body is a place

you inhabit,

it is your home

love her,

cherish her,

for she is the only one

you will ever own

— body love

Make time

for the one person

you cannot escape

— yourself

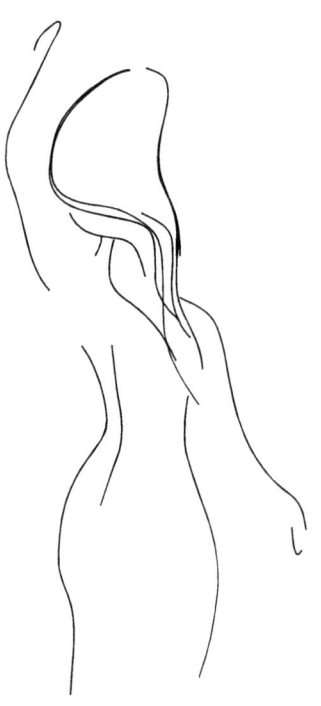

Fall in love
with the moon and stars,
with a lover whose love
is engraved on your heart

fall in love
with where you are now,
for that is all that lives

keep your world spinning
in rapture
by falling in love
a little more
with *you* each day

Grow

bloom

learn to ease through ...

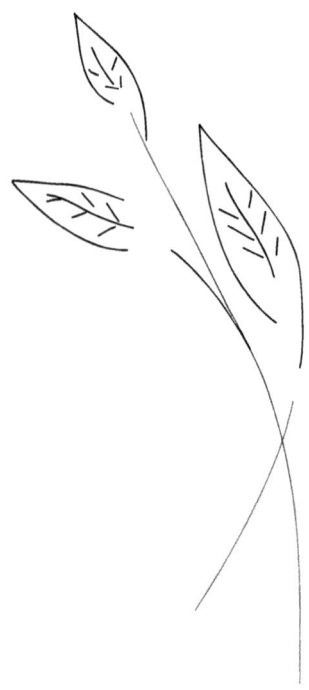

Rise from the fall
that became your fate,
do yourself justice
reclaim your space

own what has always
been yours to take,
live in your power,
reinstate your grace

let your kingdom come
and flourish high
to your rightful place

free history
and lace
your true destiny

live out loud,
breathe love,
create your kingdom
in love

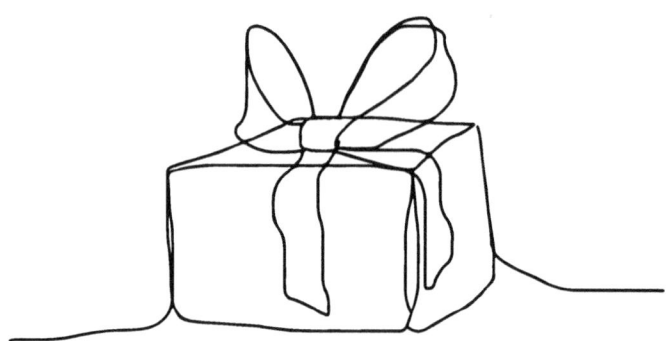

Love is a luxurious gift
we offer ourselves beyond
labels, experiences
or attachment

self-love is fearlessly loving
the essence of who you are
with conviction

silk on ice

In the illusion
the aperture of my lens
was out of focus

in the moment the floor
left the soles of my feet,
I fell through
and met divine grace

there was a first time
but never a last,
impermanence abides
an ephemeral nature

— I am listening now
more than ever,
I return home to you

whatever the world
outside myself sweeps
into my lap,
I always have me
my home
my breath
my heart
my truth
my life
is my choice,
I return to grace,
do you?

Kingdom

inner wisdom

Loving life fiercely
made impermanence known,
in the fire
I laid in torment
learning to breathe once more

between fury and flames
the mercurial nature of mind
highlights *the game*

— the satire of love
here we hunt
searching —
collecting thimbles of love
in haste,
weighing down bridges
burning away

it is time to remember
lessons of self-love
to change the inner state

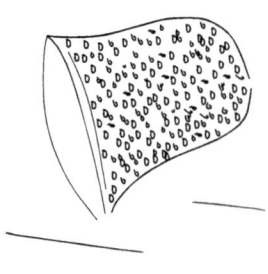

Be of faith
love and be loved
give and be given
let light be one
with your hand and heart
and you will see darkness
fall slave to its master —
be as one
with one and
peace will lay where you lie —
be the maker of your mark
and conquer lust of life
let go —
and ease will come to you
for no mortal moves to the eternal,
the immortal knows this truth —
listen to the whispers
in the depth of silence,
wisdom rests patiently
beneath your roots —
come what will
do or do not,
one golden thread will be woven
with your hand and heart,
choose love,
eternal love for all

$$\frac{Love}{Fear}$$

sian flanagan

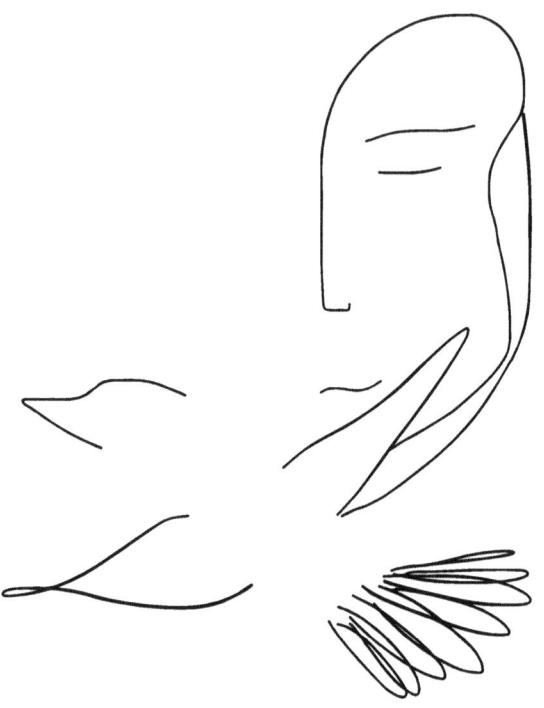

The soul owns
the land of refuge

welcome your wisdom
and you will know freedom

The beauty of grace
awaits in solitude

sian flanagan

Dwelling in negative thoughts
is like declaring war on yourself,
the battle is real
and often fatal

— words create reality

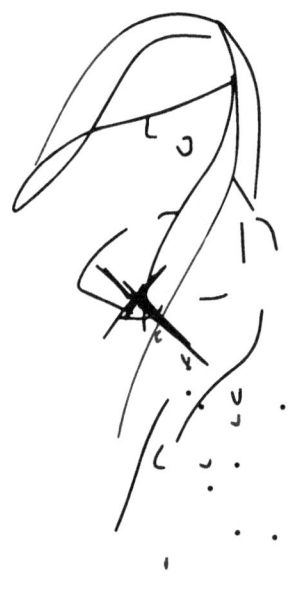

silk on ice

We must leave the mentality

we are bound to

in order to discover

who we are capable of becoming

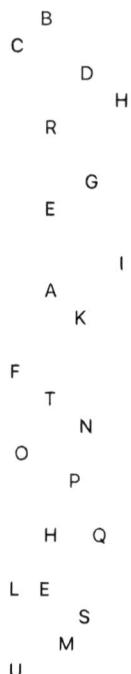

People will judge you,

people will give into their

preconceived notions of you

breathe,

opinions do not belong

to your world

Theories that we are
anything but complete
are a lie

— enough

Forgo worry
and selfish guilt
they will elude and deter you
from all that you are

— be

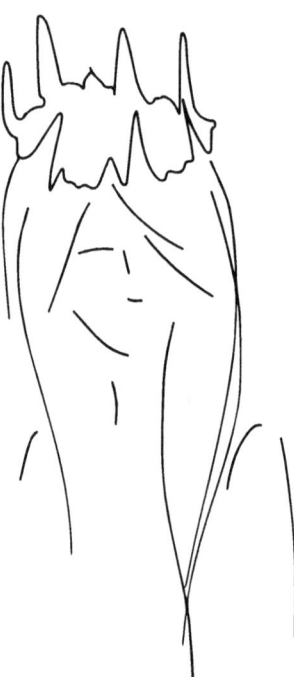

silk on ice

People will criticize you,
underestimate you
and denounce you

do not hold
what someone asks
you to carry

make a new vow
to what you will marry

sian flanagan

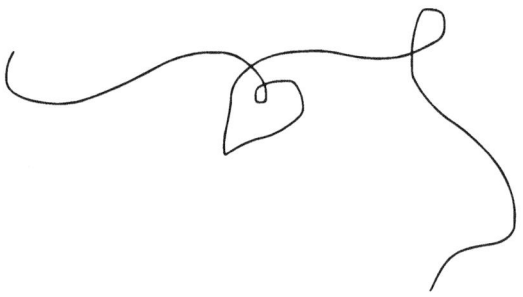

Defy the gravitational pull

in your head

and listen

to your heart instead

Hold steady
when waves form,
stillness is sure to come

there —
raise light
in darkness

find your glow
in the aftermath,
let words of wisdom
breathe into spaces
where thoughts
have left you stranded

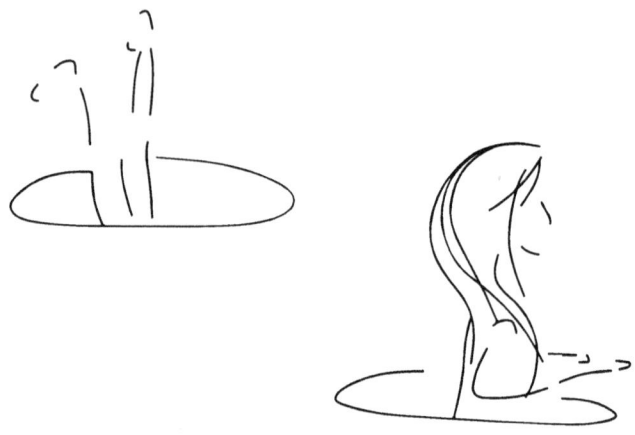

All we ever do
is think our way in
and out of things

— choices

Priorities navigate

the reins of balance,

unwind,

nourish in the bare essentials

learn how life lives naked,

the rest is smoke

lost in shadows

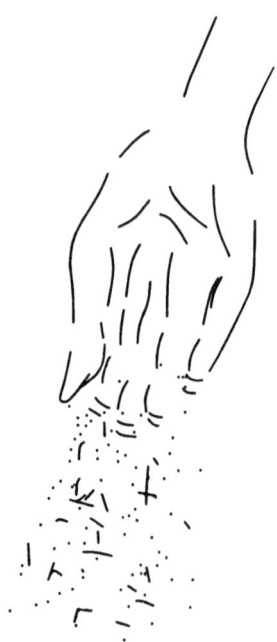

Have the courage

to empty fear

from your mind and heart

there you will learn

of your true art

Our hardest trials
call for our
greatest nature

— love

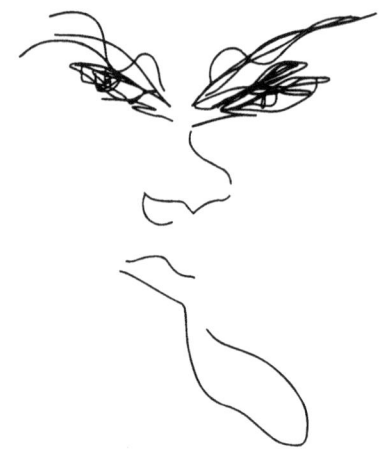

Remember

greed feeds off a mindset

full of scarcity and lack

— his neighbors are fear and ruin,

for all he knows

is what teases

and tempts his eyes

never observing

from a bird's-eye view

— and so the crumbs

he feasts on

will always be

the scraps he chews

Holding true to standards
paves deep grooves,
allowing you
to live comfortably
in your shoes

— check your moral compass
and be brave enough to erase
the faulty attributes
you hold and display
that overturn your
highest reign

— acquire knowledge
yet be wise
to keep what makes sense
and say goodbye
to what no longer applies

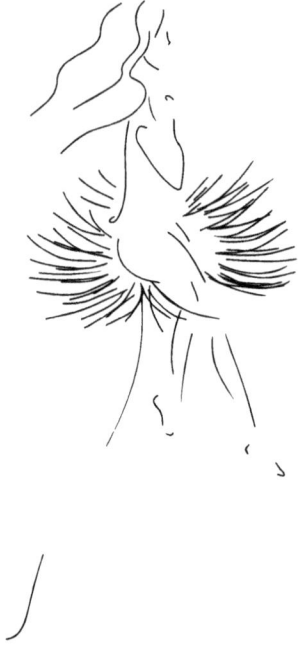

Care about the inner spark that says:

things can be different,

if I step outside

these walls of fear,

I can be free

Do not fear — fear

own it,

and it will never own you

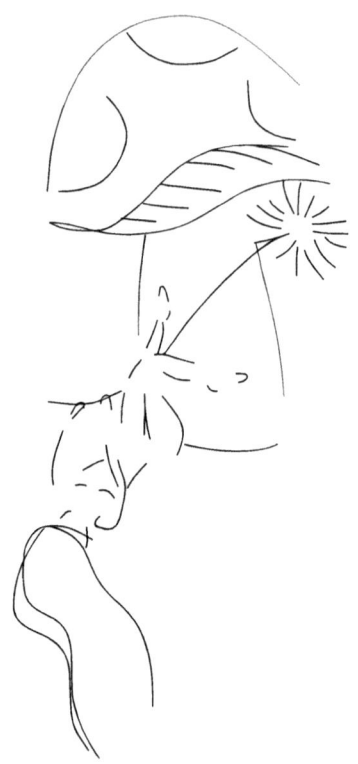

Courage is stronger than fear,
the challenge is not giving into fear
for a false sense of security

— bravery

silk on ice

Clarity is the space created
in the absence of fear

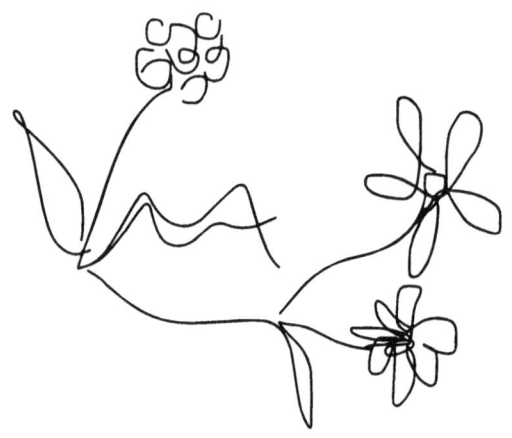

Victory is sweet
because it is painted
with the scars of pain,
sacrifice and hard work

the mark of transformation
and evolution
— fears conquered
by a loving,
soulful revolution

Diamonds are created from coal
because of the immense stress,
strain, compression and heat
applied by force ...

unite with your origin
and stretch yourself
to deepen roots of resilience
so you shine bright like a diamond

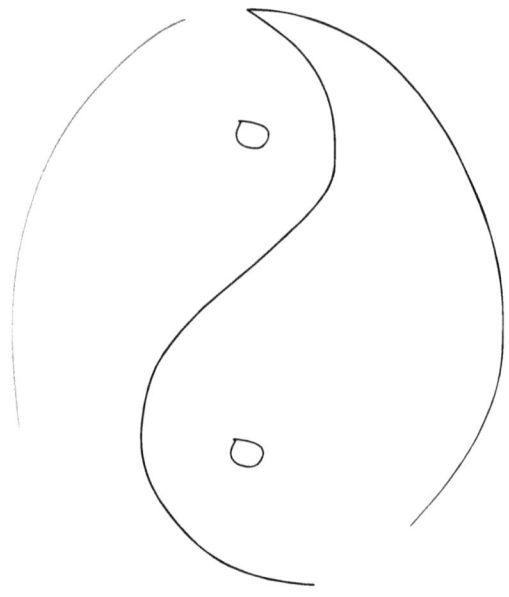

You cannot live out
your well-traveled soul
without yin and yang

Harmony always finds
a way to balance out
the master plan

karma stretching
from thoughts
to hands

dharma opening up
her cosmic cans,
driving purpose on our
earthly land

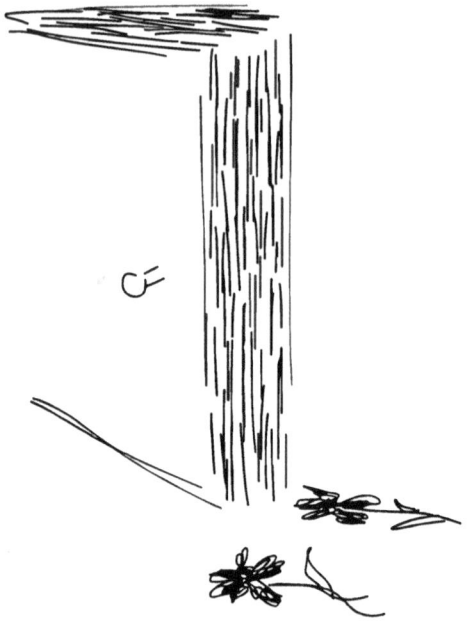

When your intuition says *no*
you must learn to honor that

— gut feelings

A neurotic mind
only sees
one side of the coin

— unconscious

Extraordinary

is tailoring words into action

by pronouncing them

as verbs

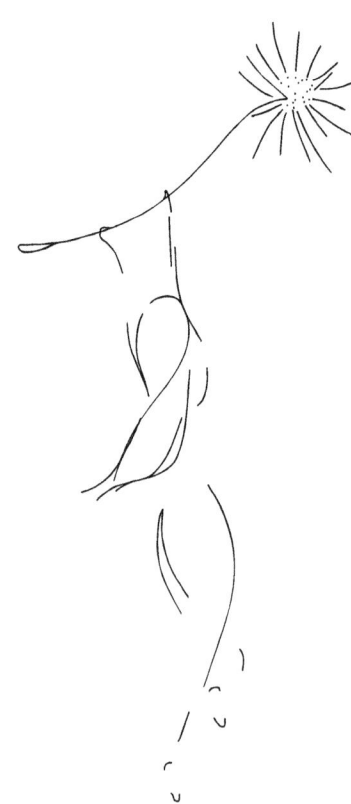

It is rare one knows
unconditional love
and support
without expectation

do not fall prey
to reptilian brain
persuasion

align with
heart-centered
meditation

We must let things

die and decay

so we can nurture the new

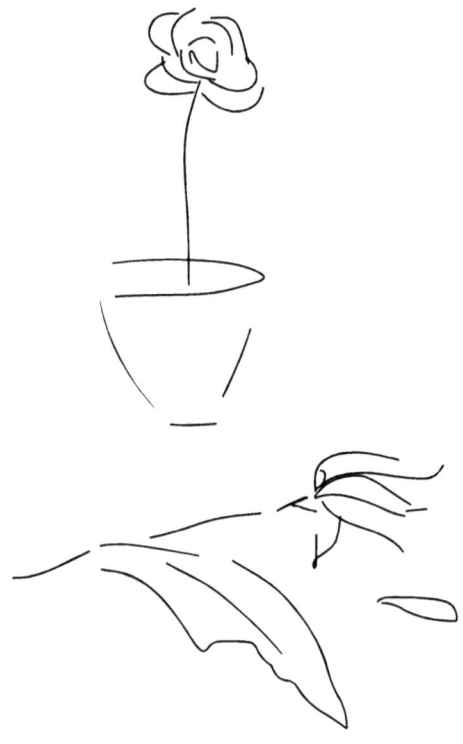

silk on ice

Logic often forms
a tension belt
— surrender

flow is the way,
the only way
that leads you effortlessly
to the destinations
you were born to pave

sian flanagan

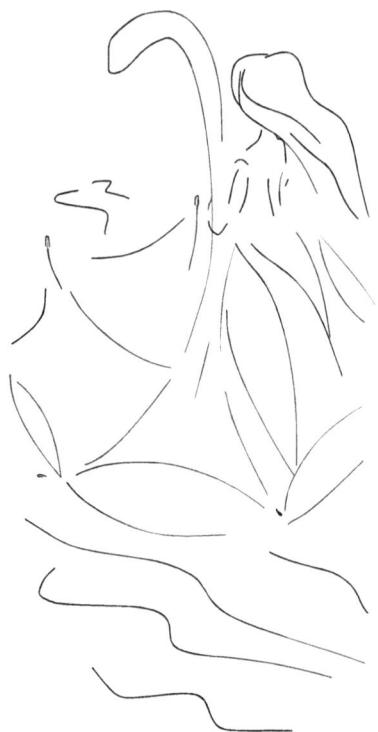

We are shadows
figures and dust
dancing in the moonlight,
wild and obscure
we go into the night
and rise with the moon

— universal truth

Flow is the language

the arcane world speaks,

you must feel her

as she moves in waves

that do not preach,

she is subtle

and sweet

like a whisper

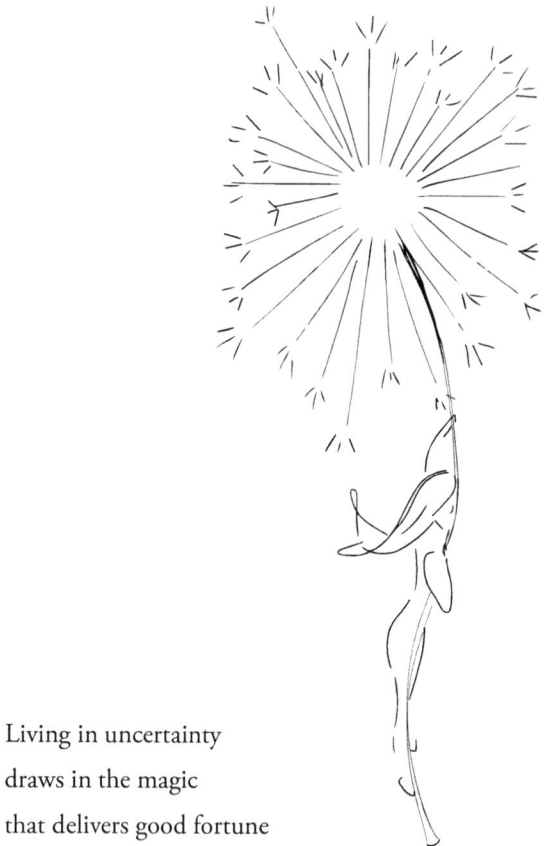

Living in uncertainty
draws in the magic
that delivers good fortune

— serendipity

The element of surprise
favors those who share
themselves and their gifts
without expectations

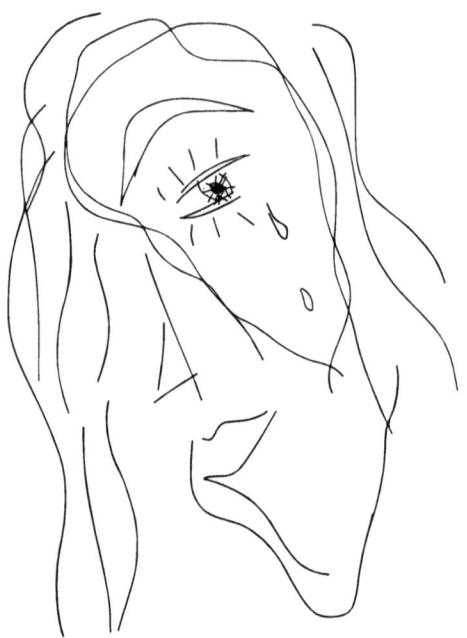

Let patience be
a timeless influence

— healing

Seasons
emotions
they are all the same
coming and going
as tides change —
nature runs
on the tips of our tongues,
down into the caverns
of our lungs,
and like common laughter
from comedic chatter,
tears too
are sentimental and natural

when salty weather
from our eyes,
hits the rug
or hand-laid tiles,
hearts fill the ocean
with tragedy and love,
feeding the collective
consciousness,
seasons change
emotions come
a natural law
we cannot outrun

Stillness

allows one

to fall in love

with the way

the world moves

— observe

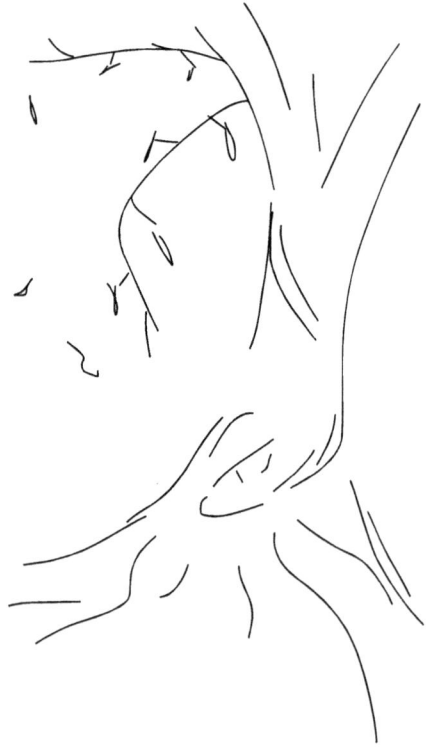

silk on ice

The process of transformation
exists everywhere
in everything
the only difference
is how we are changing

— becoming

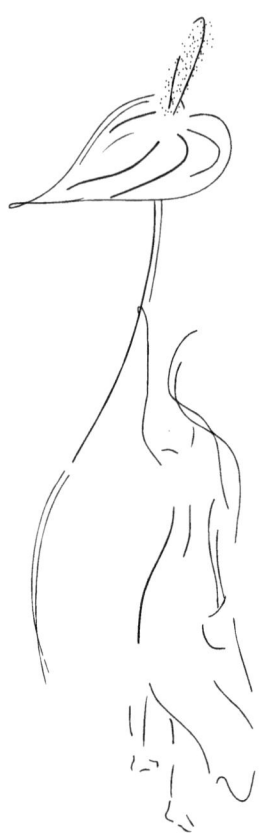

Naturalness
is the radiating force
of grace

— real

silk on ice

I never knew *her*
until I gave my heart — openly

I never knew real
until I touched
the hand of a stranger
upon soil I had never stood

I never knew real
and then I found peace in the
reflection of another's eyes

in time,
I saw us all
as one
in the mirror
of unity's smile

there,
I met real
for the first time
and I came home
with gratitude in tow

Limitless is an entry point
into the silent existence
of infinite possibility,
where no inquiry,
no yearning or thought grapples,
where all known and unknown
is fused as one

— Zen

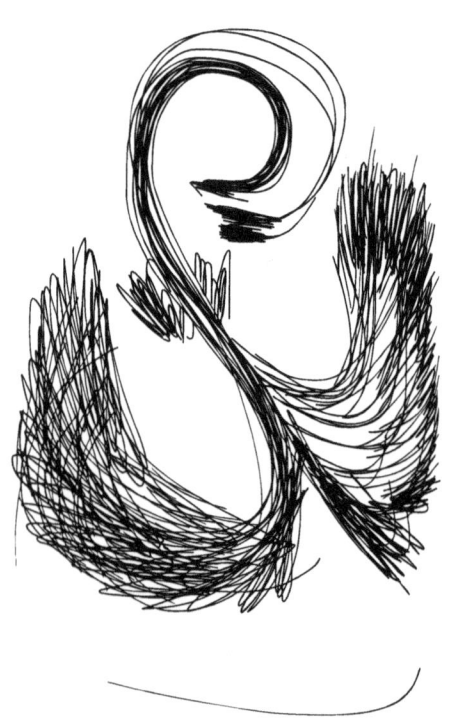

silk on ice

The whisper you hear
behind the mask
is the *wisdom*
that invites your attention

— enlightenment

Marvelous things
transpire
when you own
your space
with conviction

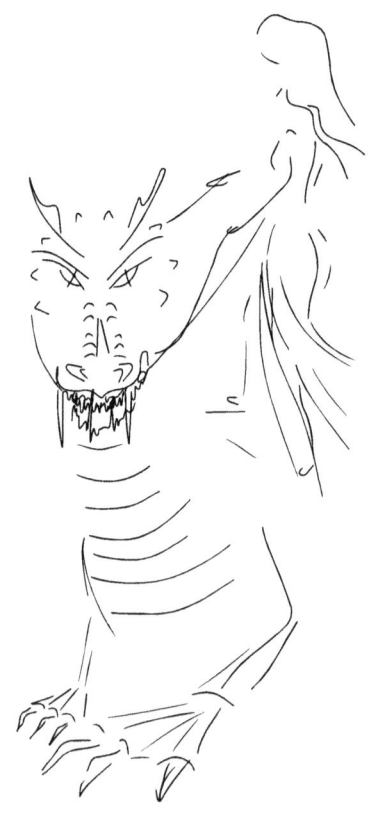

silk on ice

We are free-flowing energy
we are bound to nothing,
we are the ultimate
physical and chemical
expression of divinity

Trust is everything,
— a flower cannot grow
with ease
without trusting
rain will return

without trust,
all else fails
without trust
words hold no weight,
connection is broken,
— love distorted

and without faith
nothing blooms,
no-thing lives
where love cannot exist
in its natural state of harmony

— practice trust first,
witness the lessons
from Mother Earth

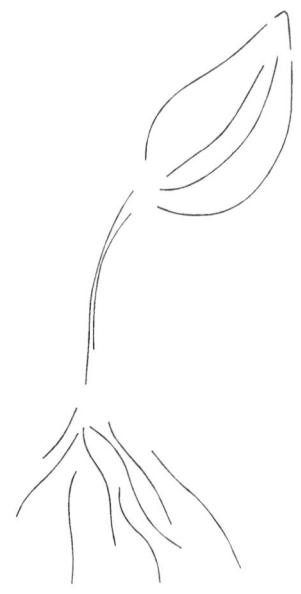

silk on ice

Trust is a bond
that seals
the eclipse of truth

What is acceptance but love of self?

what is peace but to care for all things?

what is aliveness but devotion to loving life?

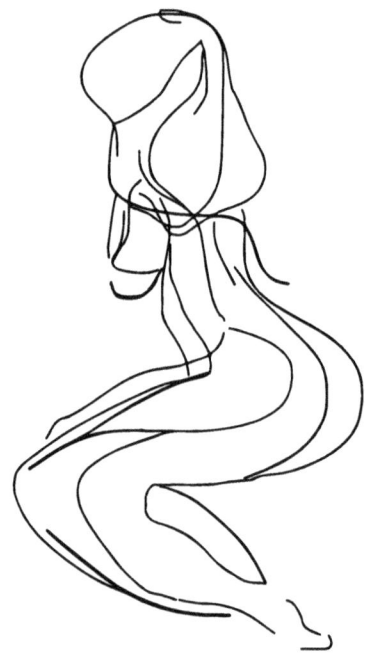

Preserve your love

by living in accordance with virtues

that emanate your liveliness

Self-love
is the birthplace of
self-esteem, confidence
and personal sovereignty,
a magnetic frontier
for new beginnings

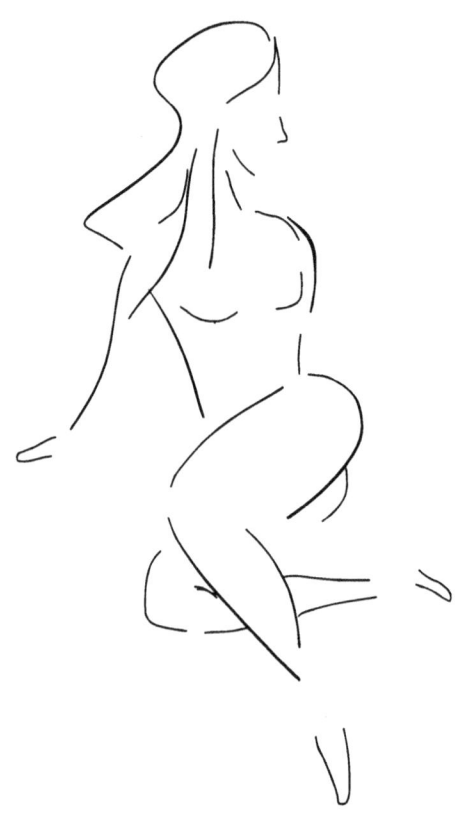

silk on ice

Only from the heart,
can we share
from a place of pristine love
and reverence

— we truly give
when we know
contribution stems
from a full cup

You know what is beautiful and rare?
a woman who values
common sense and intellect
before caring about her hair

— priorities

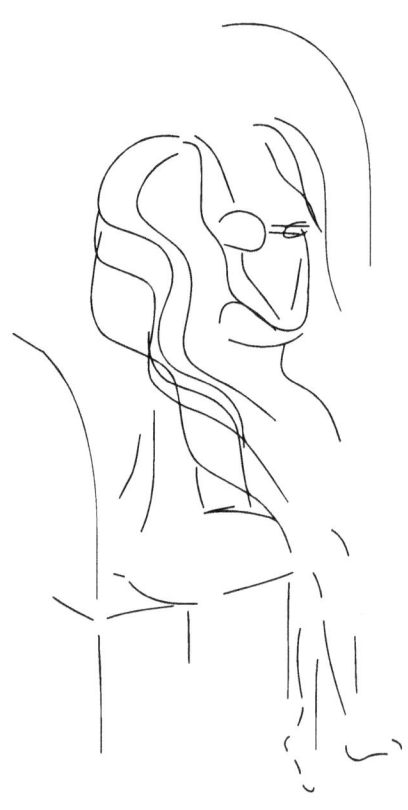

silk on ice

I value dressing my mind
with knowledge and creativity
over my body with clothes,
any day of the week

Real beauty lives
beyond flesh and bones,
vanity is the spell that keeps
us shaded from substance

— superficial

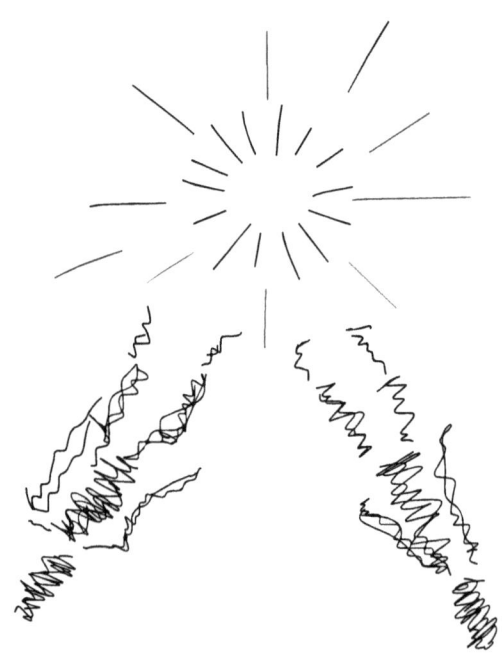

silk on ice

When the material worn
is valued more
than the mind wearing it,
we have lost all sense of real

— artificial intelligence

Fierce by day
she owns her soul
with conviction
— stiletto to toe
she walks *silk* roads,
boldly paving gold

owning her way
she wins — the game,
weaving all her pain
into grace,
tempering
her beast,
she lives
in mastery

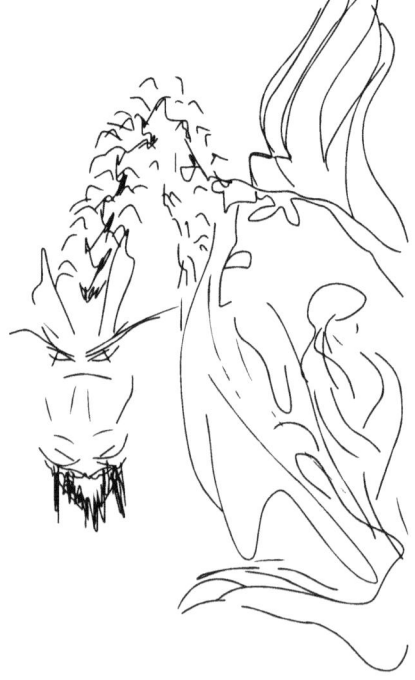

Let words of truth
strike through
victim's blame,
shine your light with
your inner flame

forgive the past
let go of pain,
release all shame,
come home to
peace at last,
you deserve
strength and
grace

let *it* be,
it's time
to set your
heart
wild and free

begin anew
swiftly

— forgive *yourself*

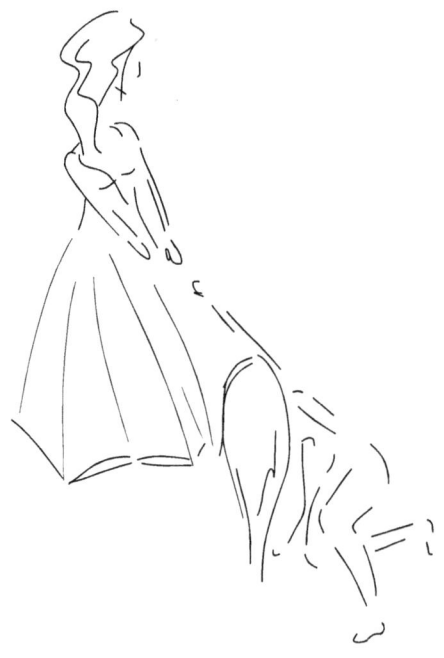

I do not need

to justify labels

or the symmetry of your face,

we are all equal —

I love you just the same,

love can be our way,

by abandoning competition

and saying hello to grace

— sisterhood

silk on ice

Take my hand
this world cannot break our bond
as easily as shoelaces come undone,
for evolution runs between us
and history shows our marks,
we are strong,
when we stand tall
in each other's arms

we are beautiful
independent of form,
independent of race
or localization,
let us commune

today hold my hand
for better or worse,
let us shred history
and make the future bright
for us and youth

You will meet your inner genius
at the gate of inspiration,
something society fails to teach

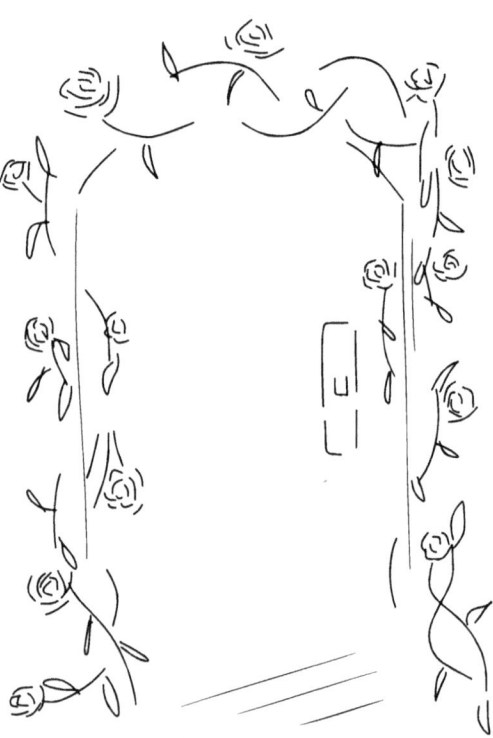

You can read all the books,
sit through expensive classes
but to study oneself
is the primary education
one must seek first
in order to know
the true nature
of one's authentic
curiosities

Intelligence merely plays

the percussion

to the master's solo

— soul

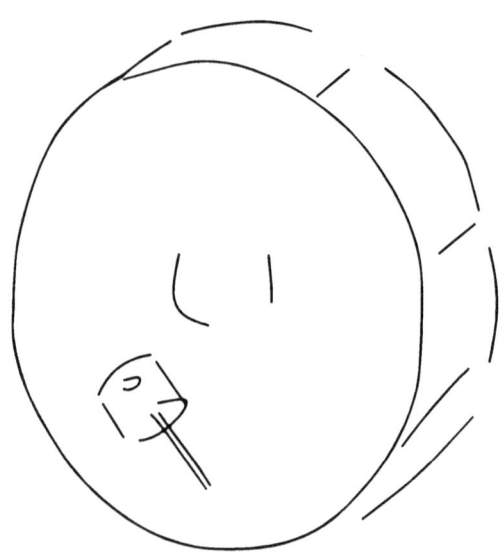

Purpose and mission

come first,

then everything else

falls into place

Your gifts radiate your beauty,
the beauty within you
is your gift

— purpose

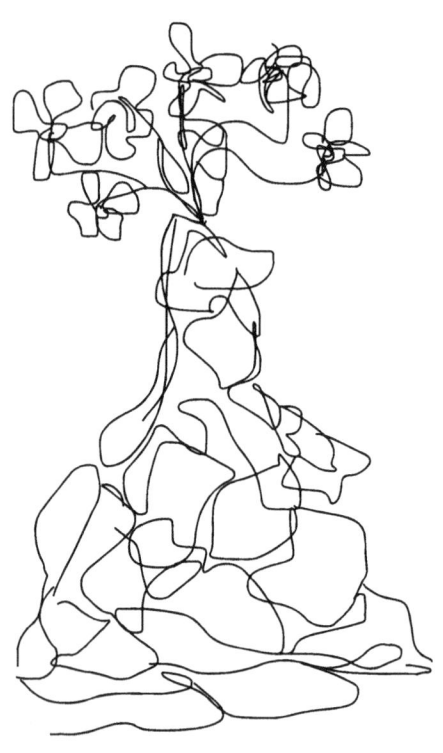

silk on ice

Allow your fervent nature

to lead your life

from the inside out

sian flanagan

Choose the colors
of the rainbow
that capture you most,
and if the rainbow
does not baffle your eyes,
walk through the forest,
and if the forest
does not appease your senses,
go to the city
and dwell in the lights

there is an entire world
for you to choose
what you wish to fall
infectiously in love with
— the choice is yours
any path is there
for you

Passion is the fuel

that magnetizes purpose

Life is full of emotional tapestries,
experiences are the flavors
that harvest seeds of wisdom
so life can reveal real fruit

— growing with truth

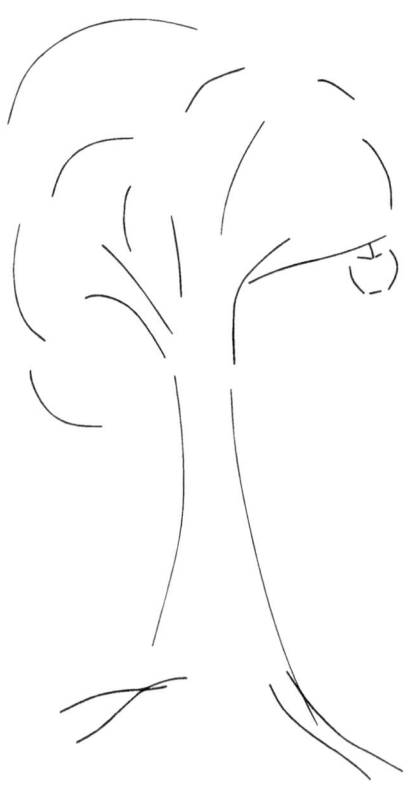

silk on ice

It is easier to live
in temporary pain
than to assault your future
with regret

— dreams

Excuses take lives
as the disease
of alibis
like a book full of lies,
a tragedy left
like a meal for a fly

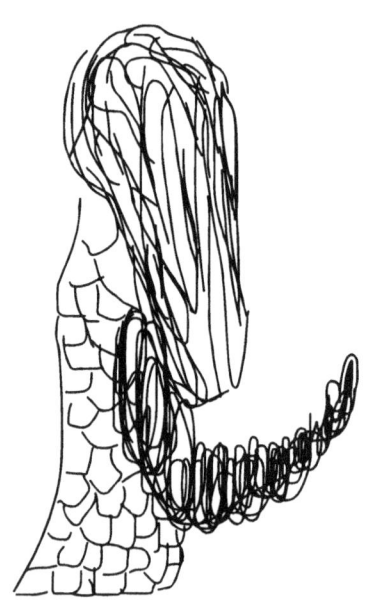

Those you admire most

cannot see

what you can see,

hold your vision

do not stray

from your mark,

visions belong to your heart

— your life is *your* art

You are a rebel with a cause
living amongst the clouds
changing form
every once in a while

here is to the free birds
with cheer and song,
here is to the free world
never let conformity
steer you wrong

sheep bow to the
lions' eyes,
keep your spirit aligned
with the rhythm
that takes you high ...

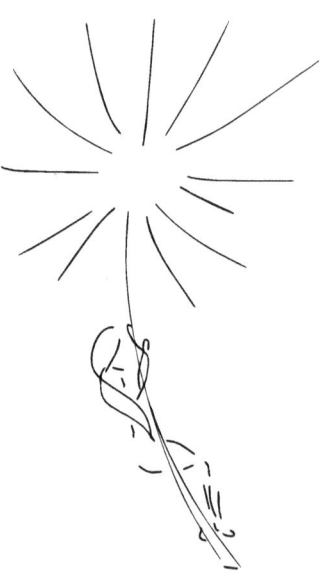

mortal one —
you know storms play riddles
be like clouds
so bones don't grow brittle,

remember love
when you feel blades of steel,
hold strong and firm
in your place on earth

come what may
always keep your soul free,
be all the shapes
you were born to be

accept your nature
like clouds
may you always be brave
and live out loud

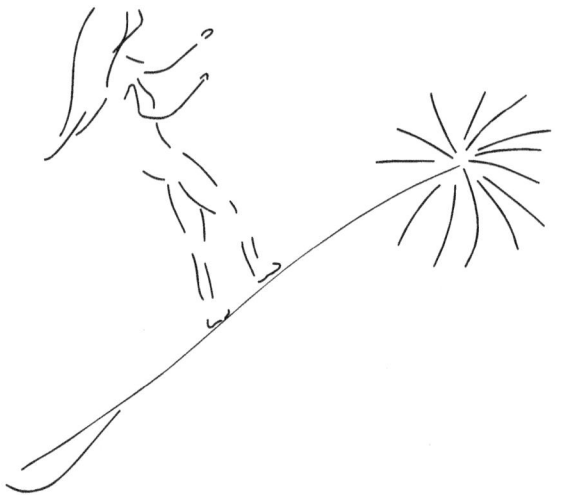

Hold goals in your mind,
embrace the unforeseen,
magnetize what you desire
by living fearlessly

— bold intentions

Do not bare a shadow
that is not yours to cast,
you already have one
trailing around with you

True power

has a calm presence

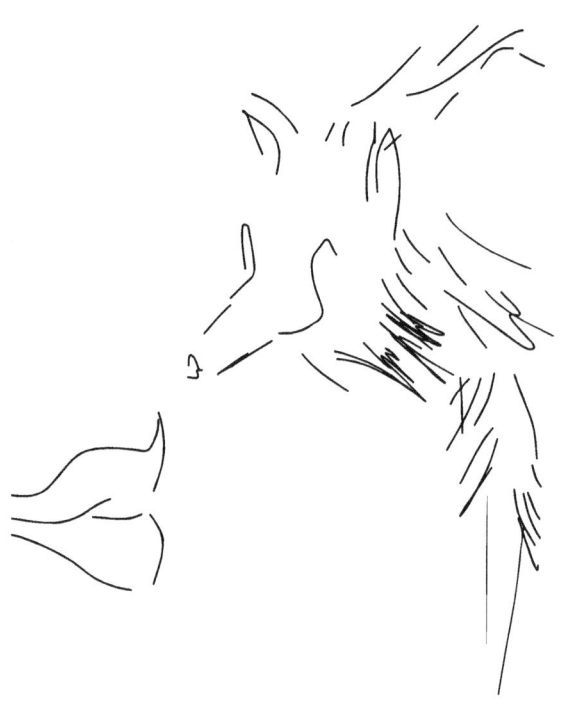

Love stems
from strong roots
and here,
beauty blooms

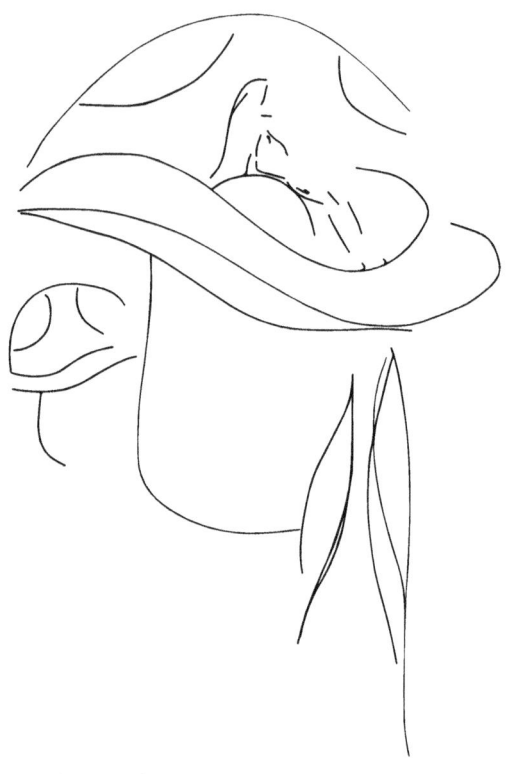

If you trace the mindset

of any great

woman or man

their origins

reside in imagination

Inspiration never dies
it lingers
deep inside

it always holds
an afterglow

waiting to rise
beyond the fence
the ego tries
to pin you behind

We have been
conditioned to believe
that there is somewhere
to be

and over there
is better
than here

— now

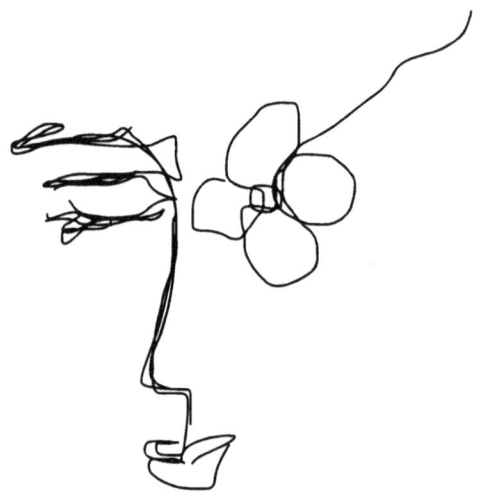

We must not forget,

the summation

of our totality

is not what we have

but rather

who we are,

who we choose to become

and the value we bring to others

— for this is the echo

we speak into eternity

Fire fuels fury
but these hands
don't play dirty,
lemonade turns
sour into sweet,
a tasteful life lives at your feet,
your story will be woven
by what you choose
to keep and greet

own who you are today
and invest
in the process
you desire to be tomorrow

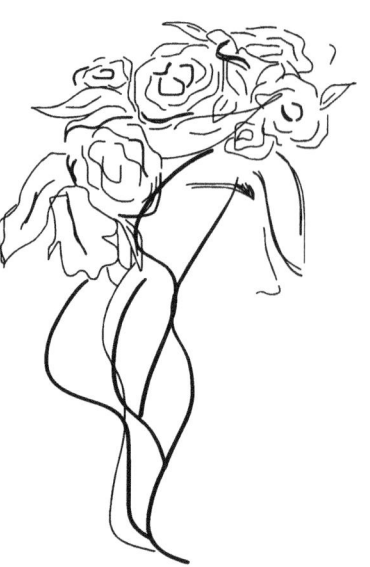

do not be swayed
by the world out there,
come home
to the land that holds
your heart,
wholesomely

— fierce love

Give up seeking love
and love will find you,
give up chasing life
and she will fall into your lap,
place this moment at the forefront
of your presence,
let go,
and you will hold again,
do nothing
and something will arrive,
surrender and you will grow
strong and wise

dissolve expectations
and freedom will be found,
invite appreciation
and magic will come around,
be curious
and *knowing* will appear,
do less
be more
in solitude
the sage comes home

The only salvation
that can save you
is taking full responsibility
for your life

independent of what lies ahead
have faith and trust
in yourself to rise

— self-love

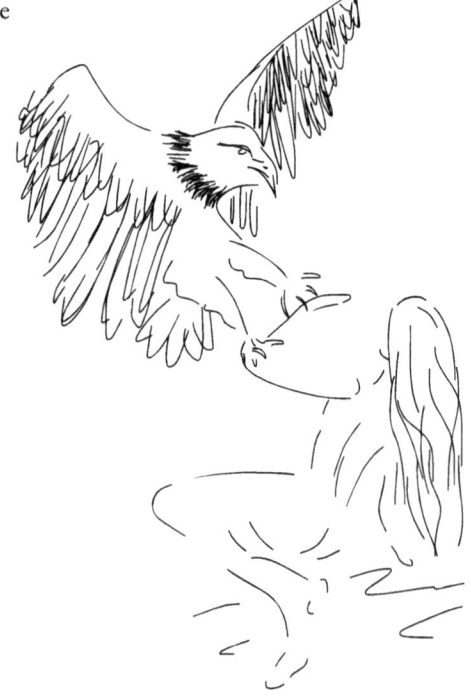

Wounds teach us
how to mend,
choices bend
the road ahead,
grounding gives us
strength to breathe,
wisdom meets us
in dark company
— *and love,*
love sets us free,
when we own
who we are fearlessly

— grace

A Note for You ...

Living in the realm of grace requires a commitment to live in a state of aliveness. Choosing to reveal your authentic self to the mirror within and the world takes courage. Owning who you are with conviction through thick and thin can be challenging, but you are worth the adventure. You are going to make mistakes, you may fail again and again, but one day you will stand and reclaim your sovereignty. So far, my personal journey has taught me how darkness holds valuable wisdom that empowers growth, if we choose it. We are human-*beings*, learning the curves of the real world. Offer yourself compassion, self-love, and patience in your practice of choosing *love over fear to know grace*. Remember, you raise your frequency when you choose love, which will outwardly change your physical reality. It is through shifting your intentions, attention, and actions daily that you begin to move from fear into love, embodying grace. *I may not know your story or your name, but I am rooting for you.*

www.sianflanagan.com
Instagram: @siandflanagan
TikTok @sianflanaganpoetry

About the Author

Sian Flanagan is a former semi-professional athlete and the founder of The Business of You Coaching. As a life, body, and business transformational coach, Sian spreads the richness of The Vibrant Living Way — a seven-step process in cultivating alignment with flow for self-actualizing authentic confidence and fulfillment. As an advocate for embodying the highest expression of self, Sian is a multidimensional entrepreneur allowing artistry to move beyond borders. She is a poet, coach, director, and founder of RantAJam Media. As an author, international award-winning short-film director, and transformational performance coach, Sian empowers entrepreneurs to embody the essence of self-love and grace to cultivate a vibrant and limitless life.

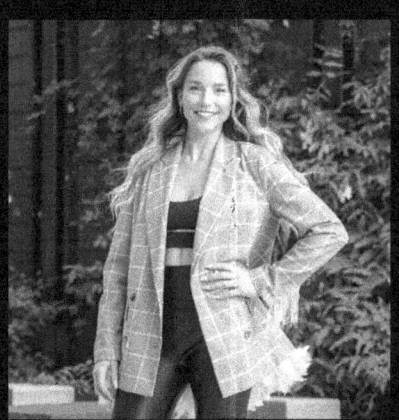

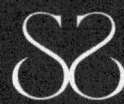

www.ingramcontent.com/pod-product-compliance
Lightning Source LLC
Chambersburg PA
CBHW051259120626
46547CB00015B/2008